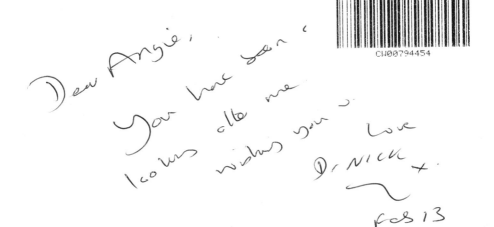

The Depression Doctor:

10 Simple Paths to Happiness

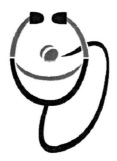

Dr Nick Krasner

For further information, freebies and contact

www.Thedepressiondoctor.com
www.drnickkrasner.com
twitter.com/DrNickKrasner

www.newgeneration-publishing.com

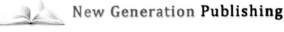 New Generation Publishing

With thanks to:

Niloo Savis, Paddy Navin, Joe Bridge, Anthony Bielinsohn, David Turner, Zana morris, Angie montout and my family.

Contents

Foreword

I have a passion for treating depression. This comes from being involved in thousands of cases of depression as a doctor and because I have suffered from it too. In the UK the family doctor deals with 80 to 90 percent of all cases of depression*. Therefore as a family doctor I believe that we are the true 'experts' of the condition especially when it is mild to moderate in severity.

My passion and expertise is fuelled by the fact that many individuals that overcome depression often became more understanding, grateful, kind and focused. In effect, however horrible depression is, it can be the catalyst in creating a great life. I have in fact heard of the term 'endarkenment', which suggests that entering into our dark spaces can be as revealing and educational as learning about our positive sides and enlightenment. This does not mean that we should become depressed deliberately, but it perhaps has a more positive function than we may at first understand. The rates of depression are so high** that one could reasonably suggest that certain levels of depressive symptoms are a normal human experience. This means it does not need to be demonized or hidden, rather we all need to work on our mental fitness in the same way we focus on our physical well being.

When I started writing this book, I had a plan. Not just to help those with depression in overcoming the condition. I wanted to teach how to maintain good mental fitness and clarity, better than before the suffering began. In other words, my aim has been to create a way to transit from depression into a happy life.

In order to achieve this I had major questions to answer. Are all depressions the same? Is the same plan for all patients likely to work, or do we need to be more specific? Are there patterns in individuals that are more likely to respond to one plan or another? Should we just use tablets or current psychological processes or are there other helpful options available?

The more I spoke with patients, the greater my conviction became that there were different types of the condition. Some depressions appeared to be more conscious based, whilst others were more subconscious in their evolution. Some depressions had a chemical cause and others were due to a lack of essential requirements. Even the ability of people to say or hear yes or no had an impact on their mental health. I plotted these and suggested a plan that was tailored to their needs. There were 10 individual classes of depression and 10 different frameworks to finding happiness. I used many available options from the worlds of medicine, psychology, spirituality and life.

I knew I was onto something when my patients were telling me that they understood their condition for the first time. They also were finding that were getting better.

Before we continue, we need some housekeeping rules. Though this book is developed to teach you about depression, mental fitness and to make you responsible for your condition, it is NOT a substitute for professional help. If you think you may have depression then you MUST SEE YOUR DOCTOR. If having read this book, you wish to change your management plan then this has to be discussed with your psychotherapist or doctor first. If you have severe symptoms of helplessness, hopelessness, suicidal thoughts or anger, then you need to contact the emergency services as soon as possible. This may be your doctor, the Samaritans, The hospital or your psychiatrist.

My work has been mainly with those suffering from mild to

moderate depression. I do believe there is much in this book for severe depressions, but their condition may need to improve first.

Another point I wish to expand on is that this book has been written anecdotally. As a scientist I am aware that further research in the future will be beneficial. However, the book sheds light on what we already know and looks at the well-known issue from a different angle. Many of the processes suggested have been studied greatly.

I do believe that however low, and for however long you have suffered depression, you can get better. Let me know how you get on at and find more information on:

www.thedepressiondoctor.com

www.drnickkrasner.com

Good luck

Dr Nick.

Dr Nick Krasner.

*49 out of 1000 patients who consulted doctor and had symptoms of depression are not recognized as depressed, mainly because they consulted for physical problems (Kisely et al 1995). Of those patients recognized to have depression only 1 in 4 or 5 are referred to secondary care (psychiatrist or psychotherapist) (Goldberg and Huxley, 1980) - this information is from Depression: management of depression in primary and secondary care national collaborating centre for mental health 2.6.1.

The Depression Doctor
10 Simple Paths to Happiness

'10 simple paths to happiness' has been created, in order to increase the understanding, the diagnosis, the grading, and the treatment of depression. It does this by re-categorizing depression into 10 new classes. This is 'The Krasner Classification of Depression', also known as 'The KCD'.

To discover your class and then severity, you can complete The KCD Questionnaire at the start of this book. Once you have completed it, all will be explained in the following chapters. You will learn all the tools necessary, from understanding your depression to loving your life.

THE KCD QUESTIONNAIRE

Answer the questions below to discover which of the 10 groups you may belong to. Then enter your results in the table below, to reveal your class or classes of The KCD.

For a **Yes**   – you score **2 points**

For a **Maybe**   – you score **1 point**

For a **No**   – you score **0 points**

GROUP 1	Yes	Maybe	No
Are you very stubborn and find that you 'just' get on with any task in hand?	2	1	0
Do you tend to take responsibility for other people's problems more than most other people do?	2	1	0
Does the word 'should' come up a lot in your thoughts and lead you to overworking?	2	1	0
Are you feeling exhausted because of all the things you are doing?	2	1	0
Do you feel guilty by saying 'NO' to other people's requests?	2	1	0
OVERALL TOTAL FOR GROUP			

GROUP 2	Yes	Maybe	No
Do you find yourself in your thoughts a lot?	2	1	0
Do others mention, or do you find, that you are rarely 'in the moment'?	2	1	0
Do you discuss the past again and again?	2	1	0
Do you think 'if only' a lot?	2	1	0
Do you find it difficult to accept a 'NO' from other people?	2	1	0
OVERALL TOTAL FOR GROUP			

GROUP 3	Yes	Maybe	No	Total
Do you feel that you are not moving forward in your life?	2	1	0	
Do you feel fearful of the future?	2	1	0	
Do you feel trapped where you are?	2	1	0	
Do others around you seem to be 'further forward' in life than you are?	2	1	0	
Do you find it hard to say 'YES' to people or opportunities?	2	1	0	
OVERALL TOTAL FOR GROUP				

GROUP 4	Yes	Maybe	No	Total
Have you lost something or someone important to you in the last 3 years?	2	1	0	
Did you suffer an episode of numbness after the loss?	2	1	0	
Did you find yourself bargaining with the world or getting angry about the loss, in the last year?	2	1	0	
Do you find it difficult to let things go?	2	1	0	
Do you find it difficult to accept a 'NO' from others or life?	2	1	0	
OVERALL TOTAL FOR GROUP				

GROUP 5	Yes	Maybe	No	Total
Do you find that you get angry very quickly?	2	1	0	
Do you find that you cannot control your emotions?	2	1	0	
Do you find that you cannot express your emotions easily?	2	1	0	
Do others say that you are emotionless?	2	1	0	
Do you believe that you have to be a stoic?	2	1	0	
OVERALL TOTAL FOR GROUP				

GROUP 6	Yes	Maybe	No	Total
Have you felt less than 100% present and functional most of your life?	2	1	0	
Do major incidents take your 'normal' low level of functioning even lower?	2	1	0	
Do you have many family members with depression?	2	1	0	
Do you respond very quickly to antidepressants but when you come off you feel low again within weeks?	2	1	0	
Do you find that your mood is low irrespective of what is happening in your life or how you think about it?	2	1	0	
OVERALL TOTAL FOR GROUP				

GROUP 7	Yes	Maybe	No	Total
Do you find that you are getting more attention from others, since you were depressed?	2	1	0	
Has your life become more secure, since you were depressed (eg more money from the government or ability not to work)?	2	1	0	
Are you worried that your depression may get better 'too' quickly?	2	1	0	
Does you level of depression alter, depending on the attention you get from others?	2	1	0	
Do you find it difficult to take responsibility in life?	2	1	0	
OVERALL TOTAL FOR GROUP				

GROUP 8	Yes	Maybe	No	Total
Do you find that you have episodes of lowness followed by an out of control high feeling?	2	1	0	
Do you feel that there are times that you can do more than is realistic in your life, followed by times of feeling that you cannot do anything?	2	1	0	
Are you confused with who you really are?	2	1	0	
Did you have a turbulent childhood?	2	1	0	
Do you have times when you find it difficult to say No to others followed by times that you find it difficult to accept No from others?	2	1	0	
OVERALL TOTAL FOR GROUP				

GROUP 9	Yes	Maybe	No	Total
Are you tired all the time?	2	1	0	
Do you find that your depression only occurs in the dark winter months?	2	1	0	
Have you found that changing your diet, has a significant improvement in your depression?	2	1	0	
Have you been having poor sleeping patterns prior to the depression?	2	1	0	
Have you been overworking?	2	1	0	
OVERALL TOTAL FOR GROUP				

GROUP 10	Yes	Maybe	No	Total
Do you have a significant illness?	2	1	0	
Have you had a large weight change recently?	2	1	0	
Are you on medication such as blood pressure pills or steroids.	2	1	0	
Do you drink more than 30 units of alcohol a week / or take illegal drugs?	2	1	0	
Have you had new or worsening physical symptoms such as chest pain, abdominal pains, shortness of breath, bowel changes, bruising, or worsening headaches?	2	1	0	
OVERALL TOTAL FOR GROUP				

Note your overall total for each group in the table below, to ascertain to which class or classes of The KCD you may belong.

GROUP	Your Score out of 10	Direction of Symptoms	Class of the KCD
		Note your overall total for each group in the table below, to ascertain to which class or classes of The KCD you may belong.	
1		Better / Worse / Same	The Mountain Mule
2		Better / Worse / Same	The Jukebox
3		Better / Worse / Same	The Stuck Trapeze
4		Better / Worse / Same	Loss Reaction
5		Better / Worse / Same	The Dynamite
6		Better / Worse / Same	Naturally Deficient
7		Better / Worse / Same	The Gravy Train
8		Better / Worse / Same	The Prince/ss and the Pauper
9		Better / Worse / Same	The Empty and Overflowing Tank
10		Better / Worse / Same	Medical
A score over 4 is significant. Which is your major Class? What does it mean? Read on to find out.			

THE KCD HAPPINESS SCORE

Answer the questions below to discover your happiness score.

Are Your Thoughts	Points Score	Your Points
Mainly negative?	0	
Slightly more negative than positive?	½	
Slightly more positive than negative?	1	
Very positive?	1½	
Blissful?	2	

Are Your Thoughts	Points Score	Your Points
Mainly about fixing the past?	0	
Slightly more about the past than the future?	½	
Slightly more about the future than the past?	1	
The future being positive?	1½	
About the present?	2	

Do You Feel You Have	Points Score	Your Points
No control over your life?	0	
Slight control over your life?	½	
Good control over your life?	1	
Great deal of control, but can give some control away?	1½	
No need for control because you feel connected to others and the universe?	2	

Do you have any physical symptoms that may be caused by or causing your depression?*	Points Score	Your Points
Severe physical symptoms?	0	
Moderate physical symptoms?	½	
Slightly physical symptoms?	1	
No symptoms at all?	1½	
No, feel in fantastic physical shape?	2	

Are Your Emotions	Points Score	Your Points
Severely negative including worthlessness, guilt, anger, hopelessness, or suicidal?	0	
Moderately negative, including worthlessness, guilt, hopelessness, or anger?	½	
Very slight negative emotions, reasonably positive ones?	1	
Mainly all positive?	1½	
Fully in your control, therefore they can be switched from negative to positive easily? You remain in a healthy happy emotional state?	2	

Today's Score - Total all the above 5 Tables' points that you have scored.	Your Points
Total	/10

*These physical symptoms may include pain, being over or under weight or physically unfit, or personal specific symptoms that occur when you are depressed, such as headaches, rashes, stomach aches or diarrhea. Alternatively, physical symptoms can include those that are related to a severe illness, such as heart disease or cancer.

PART 1
THE 10 CLASSES OF THE KRASNER CLASSIFICATION OF DEPRESSION
THE KCD

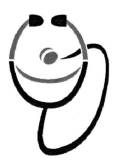

Chapter 1
The KCD

To successfully treat an individual's depression, there needs to be a specific diagnosis, which leads to an appropriate management strategy. Unfortunately, current medical practice barely differentiates one person's depression from another. Therefore, the prescribed remedies for a variety of different patients are often extremely similar. Success is limited.

'10 simple paths to happiness' and 'The Krasner Classification of Depression' (The KCD) aim to revolutionize this process. By creating 10 different categories of depression, The KCD aspires to target available treatments to the right people.

Each category of The KCD has distinct causes, symptoms and suggested treatments. Some of the classes of The KCD have their root causes in chemical imbalances, whilst others are the direct result of childhood psychological influences. A number of the groups have their foundation rooted in the subconscious, in comparison with others which are controlled by the conscious mind.

This understanding is extremely important because some available psychological processes such as Cognitive Behavioral Therapy (CBT) work on the conscious mind, whilst others such as Neuro Linguistic Programming (NLP) work on the deeper subconscious. However, certain classes of The KCD respond better to a particular lifestyle change than to either medicines or therapies.

Another goal of The KCD is to prompt medical investigations, such as blood tests, for depression, because other disease processes and lack of certain essential nutrients can be the underlying cause.

'10 simple paths to happiness' has four sections. These are:

1. Looking individually at the 10 classes of The KCD and presenting their specific symptoms, causes, and treatments.

2. Understanding how The KCD grading system works, in order to ascertain the severity of depression and to monitor an individual's mood.

3. The practical aspects, which explore deeper into areas that can affect all types of depression. These include personal boundary management, responsibility, nutritional advice, and a dozen 'tricks' for instantaneously getting out of a bad mood. Explanations about relevant psychological processes, medications and self-help ideas are also included in this section.

4. Using the knowledge from the three previous sections, the reader is facilitated in creating a personal action plan, which takes into account the individual's class and severity of The KCD.

Before I divulge the categories of The KCD, there are a few important details that I wish to address.

1. This book IS NOT A SUBSTITUTE for personal medical attention. Although this book aims to empower the reader in their understanding and management of their depression, it is fundamental that you fully discuss your symptoms with your doctor or mental health practitioner. The services of doctors will also be required for the investigation and treatment of your condition.

2. Depression is a lonely place, yet its treatment is best conquered in company. Isolation increases severity and longevity of depression, because it increases mental rumination and the sense that there is no one to help. Discussing your findings of this book with trusted friends, family, or colleagues can be extremely beneficial. They can help you uncover your symptoms, support you through creating an action plan, and share the understanding that all human beings have issues.

3. I have witnessed a dramatic improvement with many of my patients, often despite the severity or long-standing nature of their condition. Many have gone on to develop better lives than they could ever have imagined. However bad you feel today, I have great optimism that it is absolutely possible for you to achieve this goal.

4. Treat your depression with the respect it deserves. I mean it. I am not suggesting that anyone deliberately goes into depression. Yet many individuals understand themselves better and have greater compassion, empathy, and gratitude following a depressed episode. Do not fall into the trap of reproaching yourself for being depressed. Use that energy to get better.

5. The amount of time and energy people use whilst being depressed can be colossal. When those individuals learn, or choose, to use these in creating the lives that they really want, they can often do better than those that have never been depressed.

The Krasner Classification of Depression (The KCD)

Though this classification system has been devised for use by patients suffering from depression, many of the characteristics of each class can apply to mentally well individuals. Understanding The KCD and its management options can benefit everybody in creating a happier and more fulfilled life.

Below are the 10 classes of The KCD, which have been devised over the many years that I have been a family doctor in the UK. It is this role that treats most of the country's cases of depression; psychiatrists tend to only to manage the very severe forms of the illness. During this time I have treated thousands of patients with depression or depressive symptoms. I have observed that the patients themselves often recognize their own class of The KCD. When this occurs, they often feel relieved, as their symptoms are finally understood. They can then move forward with overcoming their depression.

The treatment options that are contained in The KCD have been gleaned from my knowledge of conventional medicine, psychological and self-help processes, nutrition, spirituality, and life coaching.

1. The Mountain Mule (The Struggle and the Should)

2. The Jukebox (Addicted to Sub-conscious Negative Mind Patterns)

3. The Stuck Trapeze (Life Inertia)

4. **Loss Reaction** (A Grief Reaction)

5. **The Dynamite** (Emotional Overload)

6. **Naturally Deficient** (Brain Chemical Imbalance)

7. **The Gravy Train** (Psychological Gain to Depression)

8. **The Prince/ss and the Pauper** (Conflict of Inner Child Programming)

9. **The Empty and Overflowing Tank** (Exhaustion and Deprivation of Necessities and Toxic Stress Reaction)

10. **Medical** (Associated Medical Illness)

Each of the categories of The KCD is described in depth over the next 10 chapters. **All processes mentioned in these chapters are further explored in Chapter 20 – Guide to helpful processes and therapeutic substances.** You may wish to reference this section whilst you are reading the treatments of each class of The KCD.

Chapter 2

The Mountain Mule

(The Struggle and the Should)

When Katrina (38) visited my office, she was impeccably dressed. She sat down, burst into tears for less than 10 seconds, stopped and then apologized.

"I should not be wasting your time like this," she said.

Katrina had moved to London from Greece with her parents when she was 10. At that time, her mother suffered from severe arthritis and many of her responsibilities were transferred to Katrina, who was the eldest of four children. Though her three younger brothers were married, Katrina was still single. She spent much of her time helping her family members. This had got much worse after the death of her father 3 years ago. Her mother had refused help from social services and expected Katrina to visit daily. She cooked, cleaned, and shopped for her. This left Katrina feeling resentful, but on the few occasions that she said 'NO' to her mother, she was filled with guilt. She had little time for a social life or dating.

Katrina enjoyed her work as a translator, although she felt she should do a Master's degree in language, as her boss had suggested last year. The rest of her time was spent helping the church to create their monthly magazine. She felt obliged to do this, as she had experience in writing and publishing.

Katrina's symptoms of tearfulness, worthlessness, and guilt had increased over the last 6 months.

For Katrina was exhibiting the classic symptoms of The KCD class:

1. The Mountain Mule

(The Struggle and the Should)

The common symptoms and history of this class of The KCD are:

1. Having difficult challenges, both currently and in the future.
2. Others feel that the individual is achieving amazing feats, but he/she does not share this sentiment.
3. Often the challenges that need facing are split into different areas of life, so that focusing on any one is difficult.
4. The individual has difficulty in asking for help.
5. They have the word 'SHOULD' in many of their sentences.
6. These 'SHOULDs' are predominantly 'I should.' There are far fewer 'YOU shoulds' in relation to other people's responsibility and 'IT shoulds' taking into account what a person feels life or society is meant to be like.
7. They have a feeling that only they can solve a problem.
8. They have ill defined personal boundaries; in particular, they cannot say 'NO' to others.
9. They put other people's needs in front of their own.
10. All 'SHOULDs' lead to an underlying fear that they are not good enough and that they are responsible for others.
11. Many Mountain Mules have been given too much responsibility, either emotionally or practically, as children.

Imagine a mountain mule, laden with heavy bags climbing up to the top of an enormous mountain. Inside these bags are bricks with the words 'I SHOULD' carved into them. The mule has done an amazing feat in climbing many mountains with such a load. However, it has been programmed to believe that it should do better. In fact, many of their bricks belong to others. How would the journey up the mountain be if those bricks were removed?

The underlying cause of this class of The KCD is a belief that the individual is responsible for others. This often occurs when they are forced to take on a 'parent's' role when young. They learn that they cannot say 'NO' to others. Therefore, they exhaust themselves. They become resentful of those they help, because they do not live the life that they wish to. This can eventually lead to depression, because the more the individual gives, the greater their resentment and exhaustion. There is a hopeless feeling, as their need to say 'NO' leads to guilt.

These 'SHOULDs' arise because of a subconscious inner monologue that plays in the background of their mind. This often gives the individual the beliefs that 'I am not good enough' or 'It's all up to me,' which were created in childhood. The urge to accept all these 'SHOULDs' occurs within the conscious mind. This over acceptance of responsibility can, therefore, be challenged consciously.

Most, if not all, of the 'SHOULDs' do not exist in reality. They are just self-imposed burdens. They rob a person of free choice and their ability to fully connect with others or to feel empowered. A better way for individuals to look at tasks is to choose to do them or not. There are, of course, consequences for their choices. However, the tasks are no longer punitive and when completed the individual can congratulate themselves. In this way, they get a positive feedback for their actions, instead of a feeling of resentment. Changing the mindset from a 'should' to a 'choice' also allows an individual to say 'NO.'

This act of 'SHOULDING YOURSELF'* is well recognized in psychological circles and consists of these 'I should' statements. There are also 'YOU should' statements, which are directed at others, and 'IT

26

should' statements aimed at institutions, society, or the world in general. 'The Mountain Mule' often has few 'you should' and 'it should' beliefs.

*See Chapter 20 'Guide to helpful processes and therapeutic substances' in section: 'Self help' psychological options.

Treatment of 'The Mountain Mule' class of The KCD is mainly achieved on the conscious level. Recognition that they are carrying another's burden and are punitive to themselves is a good starting point. Writing down all their beliefs of what they 'should' be doing is very valuable. These 'should lists' can run into the hundreds and thousands. Most items on the list will be 'I should' or 'I should not,' but there may be some 'you should' and 'it should' statements.

These statements need to be challenged. This again is done on the conscious level. CBT,* Byron Katie's 'The Work,'* and the 'Three Whats'* are perfect for this.

In many cases, it is not necessary to go deeper onto the subconscious. However, the fears created in childhood, which may underpin a 'SHOULD,' such as 'nobody will love me unless I say YES,' can be helped with a subconscious program such as NLP,* Inner Child Psychoanalysis,* or PsychologicalSurgery.

Another important part of treatment for 'The Mountain Mule' is the resetting of their personal boundaries, which will facilitate their ability to say 'NO.' For explanations on how this is achieved, go to 'Chapter 18 – Boundaries.'

*See Chapter 20.

I explained to Katrina that anybody taking on so much responsibility would struggle. I suggested that she write a 'should list' for our next meeting.

Her list contained over 500 'SHOULDs,' one of which was 'I should do what my mother asks of me.'

"Why?" I asked.

"Because she is old?"

"So why do you need to do everything that she asks?"

"Because she is my mother."

"So why do you need to do everything that she asks?"

"Because she says so."

"So why do you need to do everything that she asks?"

"Because...........oh, I don't know................"

Katrina went silent for a minute and then blurted out, "Because if I don't, then I am a bad person."

For Katrina, all her 'SHOULDs' led to her underlying belief that if she said 'NO' she would be a bad person. I challenged this thought.

"So if you don't do exactly what your mum wants, it means you are a bad person?"

"Yes....Well, no...but..."

Katrina underwent CBT over the coming months and challenged her 'I shoulds.' Then she went on a course, in order to work on her boundaries. She began to see that her mother needed to take responsibility over her own life. Katrina could choose to help or not. At first she felt guilty saying 'NO,' but this changed over time and her mum agreed to allow social services to help her.

Katrina chose to resign from the church paper and was surprised to find that there were plenty of people who wanted to take her place. She also chose that she would start her Master's degree in a few years' time. She went to an Inner Child Psychoanalyst on a few occasions, uncovering and challenging her underlying beliefs about herself.

She became much happier and even began dating.

Suggested strategies to help 'THE MOUNTAIN MULE' class of The KCD:

1. Take stock of all you are doing.
2. Congratulate yourself on doing so much. YOU are a SUPERMAN or SUPERWOMAN.
3. Write a 'should list':
   a. List 100+ things you are saying you should do.
   b. List of 'YOU SHOULDs' for things you feel others should do.
   c. List of 'IT SHOULDs' for how you feel the world 'should be.'
4. Challenge these 'SHOULDs' using techniques such as:
   a. CBT.
   b. LIFE coaching.
   c. The Three Whats.
   d. Byron Katie's 'The Work.'
5. For underlying beliefs from childhood, consider:
   a. Subconscious programming such as NLP or PSYCHOLOGICALSURGERY.
   b. Inner Child Psychoanalysis.
6. List your own minimum requirements in life (examples below), and prioritize them.
   a. Sleep.

     b. Diet.

     c. Time to self.

     d. Fun.

     e. Exercise.

7. Work out your boundaries with others.

     a. Read books on Boundaries or go to seminars on boundary setting.

     b. Choose for yourself how much of yourself you wish to give to others.

     c. Practice saying 'No.' It will feel uncomfortable at first, but very empowering once you get accustomed to prioritizing your own needs.

8. Permit friends, families, and colleagues to help you in your life.

Chapter 3

The Jukebox

(Addicted to Sub-conscious Negative Mind Patterns)

Mrs. Michaels did not look at me as she entered my office. She had begun speaking before she had sat down, and stared blankly at the wall as she continued.

"Doctor, my life is terrible, terrible," she said, "Oh, I don't know how I survive all the pains and problems I have. I am not sleeping and next-door's dog wakes me up early by barking. It's no good for my nerves. I feel so low and nobody listens to me."

I interrupted her flow after about five minutes. If I had not, I was sure that she would have told me that her husband and grown-up children take her for granted; for I had heard this story countless times before. She did not like the people at work and hated living in the city. Her husband had relented a few years ago and they had moved to the countryside, but she had actually hated that more and they had returned to London. She did not feel that others could grasp that her depression was worse than anybody else's. Allied to that, she could not stop eating and had put on 30 pounds over the last 2 years.

Mrs. Michaels blamed her parents for her predicament, as they had not persuaded her to abandon marrying her first husband, at 18. He had 'ruined' her because he was angry most of the time. She had then met Brent, who was a successful accountant. They had got married and had two children.

She then stared at the ground and burst into tears.

"Why did I get it all wrong, why did I move back to London?" she sobbed.

For Mrs. Michaels was exhibiting the classic symptoms of The KCD class of:

2. The Jukebox

(Addicted to Sub-conscious Negative Mind Patterns)

The common symptoms and history of this form of depression are:

1. Not being present.
2. Being self-absorbed.
3. Taking little responsibility for their life.
4. Blaming others and the 'younger self' for their current situation.
5. Recounting the same tale again and again (as if it they were playing the same CD from a jukebox).
6. Unable to focus on a positive future.
7. Trying to fix events from the past.
8. Resistance to saying 'YES' to others and to their life.
9. Difficulty recounting happy moments.
10. Inability to stop themselves recounting their tale of woe.
11. Using 'if only' a lot in their sentences.
12. Other compulsive behaviors are common, such as overeating.

The mind is like a jukebox. It has many thoughts and mind patterns that are like CDs. These are contained in the subconscious. These CDs get played again and again because the individual is addicted to them. These CDs are usually negative and they stop the person from being PRESENT.* If a person is addicted to one negative CD, then they are likely to be addicted to others. This means that compulsive behaviors such as overeating, or addiction to sex, alcohol or drugs, are common in this class of The KCD.

People with 'The Jukebox' will recount the same tale of woe again and again, to anybody who will listen. They tend to steer all conversations back to themselves and their woes. They are not fully conscious of people or their surroundings. This, of course, leads to an inability to connect with others. Not only that, but often their CD of woe is so all encompassing that it becomes a self-fulfilling prophecy.

The likely cause of this class of The KCD is the inability of the individual to become an adult. Instead, deep subconscious programs from childhood are so strong that their thought patterns are childlike. This may well have occurred if the individual's mind believes that they were harshly dealt with when younger. They have underlying inner monologues that run deep in their mind, with thoughts such as 'it's not fair,' or 'everyone thinks it is my fault.' As these individuals have not learned to take responsibility for their lives, they go back into the fantasy of negative mind patterns when they perceive something is not perfect. When life gets difficult, they spend increasing amounts of time in these thoughts. The more this CD plays in 'The Jukebox' of the mind, the less room there is for any positive thinking. This can become as addictive as an I.V. drug abuser picking up a needle.

The reason these individuals become depressed is because they believe their negative thoughts. They allow themselves to wallow and it is a downward spiral from there. People within 'The Jukebox' class of depression often find it difficult to say 'YES' to others but expect others to say 'YES' to them.

*Being PRESENT is a state of mind, whereby the individual has no thoughts interrupting the flow of the senses (hearing, seeing, feeling, touching, and smelling). In this way they can fully focus on what is happening at this very moment.

Treatment of 'The Jukebox' class of The KCD is based on overcoming the addictive nature of the condition. First, the individual needs to learn to become present. There are many examples of how this can be achieved in the chapter entitled 'Tricks for getting out of depression.' The individual needs to be able to recognize that they are in 'negative fantasy land' and to eventually focus on something else.

It is important to be targeted with the treatment of The Jukebox because therapies, such as pure counseling, that allow the person to recount their tales actually enable more of the addictive behaviors. However, Inner Child Psychoanalysis is a hugely beneficial tool in this category. This is because the underlying cause is a childlike way of handling thoughts. To change these beliefs requires going back to the moment they were created, and hence the individual's 'inner child.' It is as if there is a little boy or girl inside their heads that needs to be parented.

Therapies that access the subconscious such as NLP, hypnosis, and PSYCHOLOGICALSURGERY are ideal for reprogramming the deep negative mind patterns. This will help in reducing the addiction to them. Other processes, that over time will affect 'The Jukebox' CDs in this way, include meditations and mantras.

Emotional Freedom Technique (EFT) and Eye Movement Desensitization and Reprocessing (EMDR), which both work on the conditioned addictive responsive of the subconscious, can also be beneficial.

Learning to take responsibility and personal boundary management is also very important in the treatment of this class of The KCD. These are covered in later chapters in the book.

Mrs. Michaels underwent Inner Child Psychoanalysis. She recalled that when she was 5, she had misbehaved in the back of her mum's car, which had led to an accident. She felt so guilty because her mum was left with a limp. She began to play the accident again and again in her mind, hoping that this would stop the accident from happening. The only way the 5 year old could deal with the accident was to blame others in her head. She became addicted to this way of thinking.

Mrs. Michaels underwent hypnosis, where the 5 year old was forgiven and a new positive mind pattern was inserted.

As her mood improved, she began to take responsibility for her life. She healed her relationship with her own parents, and apologized to her husband and children for being so distant and controlling.

Mrs. Michaels joined Weight Watchers and began to curb her overeating tendencies. She also started going to the gym. Her greatest challenge was stopping herself going into her old tales of woe. She got better at this by taking three deep breaths when she realized she was in an addictive pattern. She then forced herself to focus on positive thoughts.

Suggested strategies to help 'THE JUKEBOX' class of The KCD:

1. Understand that you are suffering from an addiction.
2. Therefore, understand in some ways you are powerless to overcome this alone.

3. You will need to forgive others (especially parents) and the younger you.

4. Start to train your mind to focus on positive thoughts, even when it does not want to or it feels strange to do so.

5. Observe your thoughts, such as, 'Oh, I am complaining about the past again.'

6. Learn to say 'YES' to life and others.

7. GET HELP:
   a. Inner Child Psychoanalysis
   b. Then get it reprogrammed on the subconscious via PSYCHOLOGICALSURGERY, NLP or hypnosis.

8. Write a gratitude list every day (at least 10 things you are grateful for, even if and when you do not feel like it).

9. Do regular positive mantras.

10. Imagine you have two CDs playing in 'The Jukebox' of your mind, one happy and one sad. The more you play a happy CD, the less the negative CD plays. Eventually the negative CD will disappear. Therefore, keep focusing on positive thoughts.

11. Some people find that EFT or rapid eye movement therapies help with the addictive patterns.

12. At least three times every day bring yourself back into reality, by asking yourself, "What do I currently SEE, HEAR, FEEL, TASTE, and SMELL?"

A final note:

Post-traumatic Stress Disorder (PTSD) belongs in this class of The KCD. A life threatening or life changing event can reprogram the deep beliefs on the subconscious at any age. Treatment strategies are best focused on reprogramming the event itself. Therefore NLP, hypnosis, and PSYCHOLOGICALSURGERY can be extremely useful. Increasing evidence suggests that **Eye Movement Desensitization and Reprocessing (EMDR)** techniques are useful in war zone PTSD.

Chapter 4

The Stuck Trapeze

(Life Inertia)

Jerome, 33, slunk down in my office chair and pulled his cap down over his eyes. He did not apologize for being late. Instead he said, "Doc, you gotta help me. You gotta give me sleeping pills."

"It's me woman, she's drivin' me mad," he continued. "Me heart's been thumping, like a disco, and I ain't sleeping. You gotta help me, Doc."

Jerome had been going out with Cheryl for 8 years. She was 2 years older than him and worked as a backing singer for a well-known band. Despite some ups and downs, the relationship had been stable for many years. Then, her marriage ultimatum had completely unsettled Jerome. He had become restless, tearful, and could not focus his mind on any particular task.

Jerome also hated his job. He worked as an assistant manager for a large supermarket chain. He had considered leaving, in order to work with his brother in web publishing. Jerome was a whiz with computers but felt that this leap was too scary.

I asked Jerome if he wanted to marry Cheryl. He did not know. He thought she was a great girl, but perhaps he was not the 'marrying kind.'

"I was so happy," he said, "but now, Doc, I feel like a worthless piece of dung."

For Jerome was exhibiting the classic symptoms of The KCD class of:

3. The Stuck Trapeze

(Life Inertia)

The common symptoms and history of this form of depression are:

1. Inertia in the person's life.
2. Anxiety to move to the next stage of life.
3. Feeling stuck in their current situation.
4. Unwillingness or inability to have a leap of faith.
5. Feeling of being stuck between two lives.
6. Mind compensates for the life inertia, by causing anger or confusion.

To progress, all human beings have to jump from one stage of life to another, like artists throwing themselves from one trapeze to the next. This starts as soon as we are born. All these leaps can be very scary. Fear of the unknown can create huge anxieties, which can result in panic, confusion and ultimately depression. However, staying on the same trapeze leads to boredom, life inertia and self-destruction. This is because human beings have a need to grow and learn through their lives.

All lives require leaps of faith; from the day we go to school for the first time, to our initiation into the world of work. However, some individuals find change extremely hard. This may have been programmed into a person because of separation anxiety. Perhaps the first time they left their mum to go into school was extremely traumatic. This is particularly true if there was a close bond between mother and child.

The Stuck Trapeze sufferer refuses to jump to the next trapeze, even if it has much more to offer. Alternatively, they jump to the next trapeze but refuse to let go of the first. In this way they feel trapped and pulled by both their past and future. This causes life instability.

The reason that 'The Stuck Trapeze' becomes depressed is because their life becomes stale, which is then followed by moments of severe anxiety.

Treatment for 'The Stuck Trapeze' includes finding clarity in an individual's life and future. Is it time for that person to jump to the next trapeze of life? Plotting where that person wishes to be in 5, 10, possibly 20 years' time, helps this. Then the person makes the leap in their imagination. In this way they can find clarity and direction. Help in this area can come in the form of friends or life coaches.

Secondly, there may well be a need to address the anxiety in the first place. The fear of jumping often comes from childhood separation anxieties. To uncover this, the individual may require Inner Child Psychoanalysis or PSYCHOLOGICALSURGERY. He or she can then be reprogrammed on the subconscious via NLP, hypnosis or PSYCHOLOGICALSURGERY.

For some, simply discussing their fears with others allows them to feel safe to jump to the next trapeze. Others just leap, knowing that not making a decision is worse. Motivational speaker and author Anthony Robbins discusses this as part of his 'Pain–Pleasure Principle,' whereby individuals refuse to take initial action because of short-term pain. This reduces long-term pleasure. However, if that person really experiences the pain of not moving forward, and this becomes larger than the pain of action, then they are more likely to act.

Sometimes the best treatment for this form of depression is for the individual to just take a leap of faith; becoming present can help this.

The advice in the chapter 'Tricks for getting out of depression' may be extremely useful for this class of The KCD.

There are times when a person wishes to take a leap of faith, from one trapeze to the next, but circumstances appear to make this impossible. The individual has to consider their family, work obligations, or health. There are always some changes that they can make, even if it is only in accepting a situation; the leap of faith being in the mind rather than in action. This can be summed up by the American theologian Reinhold Niebuhr, who said, "God, grant me the serenity to accept the things I cannot change, the courage to change the things I can, and the wisdom to know the difference."

Jerome agreed with my analysis that he was scared to jump from one time of his life to the next. He then recalled that it had been the same feeling when he had started school, changed schools, went to college, started going out with Cheryl, and when he began his new job.

Jerome needed clarity to take a leap of faith, in order either to end the relationship or to move forward.

I got Jerome to imagine the life he wanted in 5 years' time. He chose being married, having children, and working in computing. I got him to cut out pictures from magazines in order to create a 'vision board' of this future. He then spent 5 minutes twice a day looking at the board and imagining what it would be like if that was his life now.

He underwent a few sessions of Inner Child Psychodynamic therapy, where he recalled an extremely emotional memory of being 6 years old and going to the zoo with his aunt. He had decided that he would wander off and see the lions by himself. When he got to their cage, he was so frightened that he burst out crying and could not move. He was alone for what felt like hours (though probably minutes) before his aunt caught up with him. This was reprogrammed on Jerome's subconscious via hypnosis.

Six months later Jerome and Cheryl were early for my appointment. Cheryl was pregnant. Jerome was extremely excited, doting on his new wife. His symptoms of depression and anxiety had gone. He had decided to take a job at a games software firm in the city.

Suggested strategies to help 'THE STUCK TRAPEZE' class of The KCD:

1. Write a list of pros and cons, for both staying where you are and your new opportunities.
2. List the long-term 'pain' you may have if you do not jump from one trapeze to the next.
3. Look at any anxiety issues of 'change' from your past.
4. Get help with keeping yourself on task with creating the life you want:
   a. Life coach.
   b. Counselor.
   c. Friends/family.
5. Subconscious reprogramming may be helpful for underlying anxiety, via processes such as hypnosis, NLP or PSYCHOLOGICALSURGERY.
6. If you cannot find the inciting moment for the anxiety, consider Inner Child Psychoanalysis.
7. Be prepared to make 'a leap of faith' in your life.
8. Learn techniques for becoming present, as discussed later in the book.

Chapter 5

Loss Reaction

(A Grief Reaction)

Janet, 42, was unusually scruffy when she came to my office. She had been feeling low and tired. She had been overeating for the last 3 months. This was the first time she had ever been depressed.

It was 6 months since Janet had lost her job at a top London accountancy firm, where she had given 'her all' for 12 years. It had felt 'like home.' The fact that her redundancy package had left her financially secure was little consolation. Janet was single but had plenty of friends and family around her.

When she first heard the news, she was in shock. She was in such denial that for the first month she would get up at 6 o'clock, ride the bus into central London and sit in a coffee shop near her old office.

She wanted to phone up her boss and offer her services for free. She went to church and mentally bargained with God that if she got her job back, she would become a better person.

As time went by she began to experience anger. She thought, "Why have they done this to me, after all my hard work?" Her anger subsided and she began to feel guilty over all the free time she had. She then felt lost and hopeless.

For Janet was exhibiting the classic symptoms of The KCD class of:

4. Loss Reaction

(A Grief Reaction)

The common symptoms and history of this form of depression in The KCD are:

1. The loss of something that is considered important.
2. Going through the stages of grief, which are shock, anguish, and then finally resolution.
3. Difficulty in creating the future, because too much focus is on the past.
4. The greater the perceived loss, the more severe and long lasting the symptoms.

A grief reaction can occur with the loss of anything, though many people believe that it is only relevant if it responds to the death of a friend or relative. This form of depression can occur over trivial or major losses. The greater the perceived loss, the deeper the symptoms are likely to be.

An individual's personality may also play an important role in the severity of the condition. People who have faith in the future can focus their attention on continuing their lives, and with support of others, often cope better with loss.

All grief reactions consist of three distinct phases:

1. An initial stage of shock or disbelief.

2. A stage of anguish.

3. A phase of resolution.

These stages were created through study of how people deal with the death of a loved one. It was first postulated in 1969 by Dr. Elisabeth

Kubler-Ross, MD in her book titled 'On Death and Dying.' She expanded the stages by splitting the anguish phase as shown below.

1. Shock or disbelief	Shock or disbelief	
2. Denial	}	
3. Bargaining	}	
4. Guilt	}	Anguish
5. Anger	}	
6. Depression	}	
7. Acceptance/hope	Resolution.	

A grief reaction can occur with any type of loss and be extremely short. An example of this can occur from as minor an event as 'losing' a car parking space. The individual sees the space and moves forward to park. A large four-wheel drive 'rudely' takes the spot. The person is speechless at first, then mutters to him or herself, 'Please don't do that.' Then they become angry. After calming themselves they rationalize that there are other spaces and they move on. If a loss reaction can occur with such a minor setback, then many past events may still be exerting a negative effect on an individual. These could include losing a job, or mourning the life that you thought you would have when younger.

Treatment for the 'Loss Reaction' can be as simple as recognizing that a person is going through the **natural stages of recovery** as shown above. Having support and love may be all that is required. Consulting counselors can be useful in allowing the person to express their feelings. Life coaches can be useful, later on in the process of grief, when a depressed stage is reached. This is because creating a new positive future may speed the recovery.

More urgent treatment may be required if the reaction is extremely severe or lasts a long time. When this happens, other underlying issues may be affecting the recovery. These may include fear of the future, total loss of the person's role in life, or loneliness. CBT may be particularly useful in helping with these issues.

The grief reaction may well precipitate other forms of depression to be activated at the same time, particularly 'The Dynamite,' 'The Jukebox,' and 'The Stuck Trapeze' classes of The KCD. Treatments for these particular classes of depression are explained in their own chapters.

Janet studied the phases of the grief reaction and realized that she had passed through five of the seven stages. She felt relieved that she would soon be in the final stage, which is that of acceptance and hope.

Her feelings, that her future was empty, were holding back her recovery. So we worked together on creating a possible future that she could be excited about. I used simple life coaching skills to achieve this. She chose that she wanted to get fit, start dating again, and start her own business.

I saw Janet 3 months later and she was looking smart in a suit. Her old boss had put her in touch with a few contacts and she had opened her own accountancy business. She was even more excited about starting to date a man that she had met through the Internet.

Suggested strategies to help a 'LOSS REACTION' class of The KCD:

1. Understand that these symptoms are part of a natural process.

2. Allow yourself to work through each stage separately.

a. Shock or disbelief – allow time to acclimatize to a new situation. Be gentle and kind to yourself.

b. Denial – discuss with others what has happened, maybe a close friend, family or a counselor.

c. Bargaining – continue to get love and support from friends and family. If bargaining for long periods, you may need to learn to become present.

d. Guilt – look at the situation from afar to get a better understanding of what happened. 'The Three Whats'* are particularly useful at this point.

   i. WHAT is happening in reality?

   ii. So WHAT?

   iii. Now WHAT?

e. Anger – allow the emotions out, either by talking or by screaming (in a safe place). Many people feel that punching a punch bag at the gym or pounding the streets for a run are extremely helpful.

f. Depression – use of life coaches and cognitive behavioral therapy are helpful, in order to start to create a new future.

g. Acceptance/hope – continue to work on your 'new' future as above.

3. If symptoms are very severe, then CBT or occasionally medication may be indicated.

4. The inability to move to the next stage of life can lead to 'The Stuck Trapeze' class of The KCD.

*'The Three Whats' are described in Chapter 16 –' Tricks for getting out of depression.'

Chapter 6

The Dynamite

(Emotional Overload)

Stan was furious that our receptionist had been rude to him. He had also argued with the traffic warden outside my office. I spent the first five minutes of his consultation calming him down.

Stan was 55 years old and worked at the assembly line of a large automotive factory. He was having anger issues, which were affecting his marriage. He had also burst into tears at work, for no apparent reason. He suffered from lower back pain and he was 60 pounds overweight.

Stan's wife had given him an ultimatum: to come and see me, or the marriage was over. The crux had come after an argument with his son had left Stan so angry that he had punched the wall. He felt ashamed of himself but blamed it on the beer he had been drinking earlier.

Stan told me he had felt like 'bursting' or 'exploding' for years. He had always held his emotions in check with either food or alcohol. He had learned this behavior from his father. He was told from an early age not to cry but to deal with things and to 'be a real man.' He recalled that when he was 7 years old, his father had smacked him really hard when he had burst out crying in front of the neighbors.

Stan had not cried at his father's, mother's or even his younger brother's funeral, but had been 'solidly there for the family.'

For Stan was exhibiting the classic symptoms of The KCD class of:

5. The Dynamite

(Emotional Overload)

The common symptoms and history of this form of depression are:

1. Uncontrolled emotions, ranging from sadness to rage.
2. A feeling that the person is going to explode.
3. Substances may be required to null emotion, such as alcohol.
4. Difficulty explaining oneself.
5. Inability to connect with others on an emotional level.
6. Being overweight can be common, as if emotion is there stored in the fat cells.
7. Physical pains manifest, especially back pain or fibromyalgia.

Through our lives, many events occur that create a range of emotions. If we release these emotions, by acknowledging them, discussing them, crying, and even screaming, they will dissipate. However, if the emotions are not released, then they will be stored in the body of an individual.

Children are allowed to cry, scream, laugh, and even rage, but this is prohibited for adults. Through social conditioning and pressure of our lives, people begin to store many emotions inside themselves, such as anger, sadness, regret, hatred, fear, and frustration.

Dynamite patients often have very blunted emotions for many years. However, at some point the emotions become too much to handle and they explode. This may occur following a minor event that raises the stored emotion to a critical level, or by one large major incident.

People suffering from this form of depression are often overweight. It is as if their emotions are trapped in their fat cells. As they improve their condition, their weight can reduce. Another common physical

49

symptom in this group of patients is that of pain, especially back pain. I believe that individuals with unresolved emotional issues hold their muscles tightly and this causes the pain. It may also lead to medical conditions such as fibromyalgia, or in some cases liver disease.

Treatment for 'The Dynamite' class of The KCD is to allow safe release of the emotion. The problem is that most patients in this class come to see the doctor after the explosion has occurred.

Release of years, if not decades, of trapped emotions takes patience and practice. An excellent therapeutic tool for this form of depression is 'The Journey Process,' where the individual's emotions are tracked back to the moment that they occurred and then cleared. This is achieved often in a semi-hypnotic state. A single session may take many hours. PSYCHOLOGICALSURGERY also uses the method of finding the emotional event and reprograms it on the subconscious.

Primal therapy can be helpful in releasing both the physical and emotional pains that are stored in the body, by re-experiencing and expressing those repressed feelings. Counselors can be useful in allowing an individual to free talk themselves through their emotions and thoughts.

As many emotional and physical pains appear to be tied together, then 'unwinding' the body slowly can release these emotional pains. I would suggest the slow restorative forms of yoga for this.

Other options of emotional release include: boxing, exercise, walking in the mountains, and writing letters to those with whom you have an association of long standing upsets. It is in the writing of the letter that the emotion is released. In most cases, it is better to destroy than to send the letters.

I believe that in many people, emotion is stored in fat cells and muscles. Therefore, losing weight can be a therapeutic emotional journey. Forums such as Weight Watchers or Overeaters Anonymous can be extremely helpful.

I explained to Stan about his form of depression and the options available to help. He concluded that going to see a counselor and starting to exercise suited his personality best.

During his sessions with the counselor, he began to understand the destructive nature of holding onto his emotions. He also allowed himself to be vulnerable and cry. He continued to find it difficult to fully clear these emotions, and was persuaded to do The Journey process. He went back and reconnected with his father. He bravely forgave his father for training him to avoid emotional release. In further sessions, he cleared many emotional blocks.

Stan noticed that as he progressed emotionally, his weight began to drop. He stopped craving food all the time. His back pain reduced also, which spurred him on to increase his exercise and to lose more weight.

Stan and his wife set aside a half hour a week to discuss how both of them were coping. It gave Stan a time to release any pent-up concerns from the week.

Eventually Stan stopped his drinking, and every time he came to see me he appeared lighter and more jovial.

Suggested strategies to help 'THE DYNAMITE' class of The KCD:

1. Acknowledge that you have emotional issues.
2. Consider emotional workshops or treatments such as:
    a. The Journey Process
    b. Counseling

c. Primal scream therapy

d. PSYCHOLOGICALSURGERY.

3. Find a safe place to dispel emotions such as anger such as:

   a. Boxing ring

   b. Yoga

   c. Gymnasium

   d. Climbing mountains.

4. Treat physical pains.

5. Lose weight, if necessary.

6. Write a letter to those with whom you are angry, expressing this emotion. DO NOT send it.

7. Reduce substance use, with appropriate help from doctors or clinics.

Chapter 7

Naturally Deficient

(Brain Chemical Imbalance)

I first met Harry P at a dinner party; to all outward appearances he had the perfect life. He had a beautiful wife, a successful business; he was fit and healthy and had launched a charity for under privileged kids in his area. He laughed, made jokes, and socialized easily. In fact, his mere presence filled the room with joy.

It was, therefore, a great surprise when a week later he came to my office wanting to discuss his depression. He had never felt 100% happy, and struggled to keep functioning. He exercised and meditated daily.

I questioned him about his life. Was he happy with his wife? Yes. Was his business going well? Extremely. Were his children well? Very.

"I know it seems I am making up this depression," he said, "but it is there, constantly."

Harry's symptoms of mental cloudiness and episodes of crying worsened with age. He first noticed them in his teens, when he was stressed about his exams. His mum and sister also suffered from depression.

Harry's outlook on life was excellent. He felt grateful, loving, and connected to his family. He practiced meditation and kept very fit. When difficult periods occurred in his life, he dealt with them fully and moved forward. However, if he did not exercise for a week he felt extremely low and sluggish.

Harry had been on antidepressants three times in his life. Each time they had worked within days, he had no side effects, and he had begun to feel 'normal.' He did not want to get 'addicted' to them and take them for the rest of his life.

For Harry was exhibiting the classic symptoms of The KCD class of:

6. Naturally Deficient
(Brain Chemical Imbalance)

The common symptoms and history of this form of depression are:

1. Family history of depression.
2. Feeling low, despite positive views of life.
3. Depression often starting in teens and getting worse from young adult onwards.
4. Rarely feeling 100% 'normal.'
5. When something stressful happens, the person enters into helplessness quickly.
6. Symptoms worsening with lack of exercise.
7. Symptoms worsening with poor diet.
8. Symptoms worsen with poor sun exposure.
9. Use of antidepressants improves symptoms within days.
10. Coming off antidepressants, the individual returns to depressed state within weeks to months.

This form of depression occurs because the chemicals in the brain which regulate mood are naturally low for that individual. The main chemical that has been shown to elevate mood is called **serotonin**. Low levels of serotonin are associated with depression.

If we analyze the levels of any body chemical in a large group of individuals, there will always be those with high, those with low, and the majority with mid range levels. It would appear to be the same with serotonin. Therefore, about 2.5% of a population will naturally have low levels of serotonin. An exact cause of why one person has a low serotonin level through their lives is unknown, though genetic causes are likely.

I have found that a large number of people with this form of depression have an excellent outlook on life. If it were not for the naturally low level of serotonin, they would be extremely happy. However, for many years they have never felt 100%. They feel 80% or so on most days. The something happens or they overwork and they go down to 60% or 50% 'functional.' They are particularly prone to Seasonal Affective Disorder (SAD).

It is currently impossible to measure serotonin levels in an individual, as the chemical stays within the brain. The symptoms of this form of depression are sufficient to make the diagnosis. Also helpful is the patient's response to antidepressants in alleviating the symptoms.

All 10 classes of depression in The KCD can benefit from serotonin-increasing medication. However, this is the only class that 'needs' medication.

Treatment for the 'Naturally Deficient' sufferer is long-term replacement of serotonin. The most usual way for this to occur is with a class of drugs that prevent the serotonin being broken down in the brain and therefore increase its concentration. These drugs are known as 'selective serotonin reuptake inhibitors' or 'SSRIs'; the most well-known of these include drugs such as Prozac, Seroxat, venlaflaxine, and citalopram.

People with this naturally low serotonin level need long-term, and often lifelong, serotonin replacement.

Because the brain has been so starved of serotonin in this class of depression, I find that treatment with an SSRI can work within days. Most literature looking at all forms of depression suggest that the SSRIs take 3–4 weeks to start working. I like to use longer acting SSRIs in this group if possible (such as fluoxetine) so that if there is a missed pill the symptoms do not return. Also this group may benefit from titrating the dose. The normal dose may be 20mg a day for fluoxetine, but may cause slight side effects (e.g., blunting of emotions or poor sex drive), but by reducing slightly this may overcome the problem. Sometimes I get my patients to take a full tablet most days but then half a tablet twice a week.

Other chemicals have been shown to help in raising serotonin levels. These include over the counter remedies such as St. John's Wort and 5HT.

All therapeutic substances are discussed further in Chapter 20. All have potential side effects and therefore are best prescribed, or discussed, with your doctor before commencement.

When Harry recognized that his condition was purely chemical, he accepted that lifelong medication was the way forward. He recalled that when he took a pill he was good, and when he did not his mood would get worse. He also began to understand that he was not becoming addicted to the medication, but that as it worked well he felt better.

I was invited to his spacious home for another dinner party a few weeks later and Harry told me how great he was feeling. Despite my warnings, he had not had any side effects from the medication.

Suggested strategies to help the 'NATURALLY DEFICIENT' class of The KCD:

1. Need to see doctor for treatment.
2. SSRIs likely the best drugs of choice.
3. Herbal medication may be useful such as 5HT, St. John's Wort, or SAM-E.
4. Understand that this form of depression is chemical and 'out of your control.'
5. Allow yourself to go on long-term replacement therapy.
6. Medication to be increased if necessary, until symptoms improve, as long as there are no side effects.
7. If necessary, titrate dose up or down to desired effect with help of your doctor.
8. If coming off long-term therapy, reduce slowly and if symptoms recur, go back on old dose of therapy.
9. Regular exercise.
10. A balanced healthy diet.
11. Sunlight.
12. Multivitamins are useful, especially including B complex.

Chapter 8

The Gravy Train

(Psychological Gain to Depression)

Geeta, 39, was curled up in her bed. She clutched onto the blankets tightly and only occasionally peeked over them to look at me.

I had been asked to visit her house, as an emergency situation had occurred. Geeta had threatened to kill herself. This had occurred after her husband had left for an extended business trip.

Her husband's attentive family surrounded Geeta. Her original family lived in Pakistan. She had left her family to marry when she was 18. She had four children, the eldest of whom was leaving home in a few weeks in order to study medicine.

Suddenly her husband burst into the room, having cancelled his business trip. He sat by her side as Geeta spoke.

Geeta told us both how helpless she felt. She did not know what had come over her when she had threatened suicide, but felt those symptoms regularly. She was exhausted and confused. She needed more help. This was despite having a maid and her mother-in-law, who helped with the children. She also wondered if she had a serious medical complaint.

Her husband was not giving her enough attention. He was spending all his time working in the family shop. She also felt abandoned by her son, who was about to start university. She had a very close relationship with him. She also hated her mother-in-law's constant criticism of how she ran the home.

For Geeta was exhibiting the classic symptoms of The KCD class of:

7. The Gravy Train
(Psychological Gain to Depression)

The common symptoms and history of this form of depression are:

1. Helplessness.
2. Situation improved by changes of behavior of others towards the affected.
3. Difficulty in accepting other people's decisions or behaviors.
4. Drama affecting many people.
5. A lot of help being given to the depressed person.
6. Symptoms getting better with help but reverse if help taken away.
7. Inability of others to break free from the depressed person.
8. An inability to hear 'NO' from others.
9. Obvious psychological gains available, such as:
    a. Being off sick from work or being looked after by the State.
    b. Keeping hold of family members.
    c. Avoiding responsibility for past actions.
    d. Hurting others, so they understand the individual's pain.
    e. Getting financial and logistical support for things that are the person's responsibility.

Depression can be a very powerful tool. It affects not only the individual but also those around that person. Severe depression, especially if suicide is threatened, can alter a whole family's behavior.

The 'sufferer' may receive more attention, help, understanding or forgiveness for his or her own decorum.

In fact, depression and suicidal suggestion can be used to manipulate others.* It works by either facilitating others' feelings of guilt or fear of loss. Depression can also give the sufferer an excuse for avoiding personal responsibility.

*Suicidal thoughts and suggestions can signal deterioration in a depressed person's condition. It may also lead to a suicide attempt. Therefore it is vital , if you or someone else has suicidal thoughts, suggestions, or actions, to get medical help straight away.

In general, 'The Gravy Train' can benefit an individual by:
1. Increase in attention.
2. Being the victim –'It's not my fault, there is nothing I can do about it.'
3. Causing pain in others. This is especially common in children of all ages. A depressed person may make a parent feel inadequate and guilty.
4. Getting time off work/life.
5. Using Depression to mitigate failure.
6. Keeping control of people, such as preventing a partner from leaving.

In many cases of 'The Gravy Train,' the individual is not conscious of the manipulation that they are exhibiting. They often feel that they have no power. It is often the sub-conscious that creates the scenario, as the best solution to a certain situation.

One of the most telling signs of this form of depression is that the drama affects many people. When the individual receives the actions or responses that they want, their depression often improves. When the help is taken away, their depression gets worse. In this way, the individual keeps control of people around them.

'The Gravy Train' sufferer has underlying fears, which causes their behavior. These fears include that of being lonely, poor, or inadequate. They cannot cope alone. Their manipulation has often been learnt over years.

They can often have boundary issues, which are: they cannot accept a 'No' from others and cannot say 'Yes' to others and life.

Treatment of 'The Gravy Train' class of The KCD needs to incorporate the entire family dynamics. For the individual is enabled by good meaning friends and family to continue their manipulation. Those around the individual may feel guilty and hence obligated to help. This aid often makes the situation continue and rewards the depressive symptoms. The sufferer will not get better until the enabling stops. **Therefore, to stop the depression the enabling must cease.**

The manipulation is often done expertly so that professional help is vital in forming a plan against it. In many cases a psychiatric team is required to help the family in forming a 'safe' strategy. Family therapy can give an ideal opportunity for the sufferer to communicate their needs. It also allows the whole family to bond together and to understand each other.

The individual needs to learn to take responsibility for him or herself. They also require new boundary settings, where they are able to hear a 'No' and say 'Yes' to others. These issues are discussed in their relevant chapters later in the book.

Inner Child Psychoanalysis is an excellent therapy for those patients that wish to overcome their depression. It will uncover the causes of fear and lack of self-belief that these individuals have. PSYCHOLOGICALSURGERY, NLP, and hypnosis can help in reprogramming the underlying feeling of loneliness.

Suicidal attempts and suggestions may well be part of the manipulation. In my experience, those in this form of depression do not commit suicide. However, the situation requires the intensive help of an experienced health professional, in order to guide the family in managing the situation.

With the help of a local psychiatrist, a strategy for all the family was enforced. It was agreed that positive reinforcement for provoking multiple crisis be avoided. Instead, a contract was created whereby Geeta gained the attention she required from her husband and son. She would lose attention for 'acting out' in a helpless manner.

Part of the contract included Geeta going for Inner Child Psychodynamic treatment to look at her subconscious fears.

During psychoanalysis it was revealed that she had a fundamental fear of abandonment. This occurred at the age of 3, when she was alone in her room during a storm. This was reprogrammed using a hypnotic approach.

In return for going to psychoanalysis, her husband agreed to attend family therapy.

Suggested strategies to help 'THE GRAVY TRAIN' class of The KCD:
1. An expert is required in guiding the entire family.
2. Stop positive reinforcement of dramatic behavior.

3. Family therapy is useful, in order for the individual to be 'heard.'

4. Family therapy, as whole family is affected.

5. Boundary issues need to be worked on, so individual can hear 'NO' and say 'YES.'

6. Psychotherapy to reveal underlying fears.

7. Subconscious reprogramming of fears via hypnosis, NLP or PSYCHOLOGICALSURGERY.

8. Individual needs to learn to take personal responsibility.

9. Remove psychological or physical gain to being depressed.

10. A contract can be drawn up, in order to reinforce healthy behavior.

Chapter 9

The Prince/ss and the Pauper

(Conflict of Inner Child Programming)

Mrs. Fazakerly was a 70 year old lady who could discuss high-level quantum mechanics or Carl Jung for hours. She lived alone and was a retired schoolteacher. Her life had been plagued by her vacillating mood. One day she would be over-excited, and the next she could feel depressed and helpless. This had got worse with age. Our facility had experienced her moods for years. Some days she would argue with staff, whilst other times she would be over-friendly.

Mrs. Fazakerly grew up in London, in a very loving home. Her mum had treated her like 'a prince/ss.' Unfortunately, as London was plunged into the Second World War, she was sent away to the 'safety' of the countryside with her brother. She was 5 years old. Her new guardian, a Mrs. Johnson, was an extreme disciplinarian. She would shout and occasionally hit the children. If they misbehaved they would go to bed starving. She felt like 'a pauper.'

Mrs. Fazakerly had been married twice, both times to an abusive partner. She had been single for the last 30 years. She had been admitted four times into mental health institutions between 1965 and 1985. She was diagnosed as suffering from manic depression (now termed 'bipolar disorder'). She was treated with strong medication, including lithium. When she remained on them, her condition was more stable.

When she was low, she felt that she should be doing better in her life. She had an unnerving sense that she should be helping others, and did not deserve the small house that she owned. During her manic phase she felt totally disconnected from reality. It was as if her whole existence was being played out in her head. She became addicted to her thoughts, 'that she was the center of the world.'

It was as if Mrs. Fazakerly had two distinct personalities: one that was down and hard on herself and exhibiting symptoms of 'The Mountain Mule'; the other was self-centered, manic and addicted to her thoughts, leading to a likely diagnosis of 'The Jukebox' class of The KCD.

For Mrs. Fazakerly was exhibiting the classic symptoms of The KCD of:

8. The Prince/ss and the Pauper
(Conflict of Inner Child Programming)

The common symptoms and history of this form of depression are:

1. Episodes of deep sadness and episodes of mania.
2. Inability to control these episodes.
3. There are times of feeling 'normal,' but this can be easily disrupted by minor events.
4. Feeling as if there are two distinct people in their head.
5. Each personality has a different class of The KCD.
6. These classes are likely to be 'The Mountain Mule' and 'The Jukebox'.
7. Their childhood is often filled with inconsistent messages. Hence their immature mind cannot create a single persona to account for these experiences.

'The Prince/ss and the Pauper' is a severe form of depression. It is characterized by episodes of mania followed by deep depression. These are the florid behavior patterns of two distinct personalities. One personality is often addicted to grandiose thoughts about themselves, and is termed 'The Prince/ss,' whilst the other is depressed, lonely, and feels poor, which I term 'The Pauper.' The former is often suffering from 'The Jukebox' class of depression, as opposed to the latter, which exhibits many symptoms of 'The Mountain Mule.'

This condition, which is referred to as bipolar disorder by medical professions, has many similar factors to the Mark Twain book 'The Prince and the Pauper.'

1. There are two distinct characters.
2. Each character has a completely different experience of growing up.
3. Each character has a different belief structure.
4. Each character mistrusts the other.
5. Each individual needs to change his or her belief structure separately.
6. When each trusts the other, there is a lifelong friendship.
7. The friendship is the halfway house, between the two extremes of behavior.

As children we learn about who we are. This is achieved by making an opinion about what is happening around us. From these opinions, the child's mind finds a personality that fits logically. However, if the child has been subjected to wildly opposing messages about themselves, then the mind cannot create a single personal belief structure. The result is two separate 'personalities.'

Each personality fights with the other for attention. The strongest personality wins. Therefore, each side of the individual exaggerates their behavior. One becomes good, whilst the other becomes bad. One is a giver and the other a taker. One is depressed and the other manic. Each personality becomes so polarized that neither can fully connect with other human beings.

Treatment for 'The Prince/ss and the Pauper' class of The KCD can include:

1. Each personality is to be treated separately.

2. Both will require in depth Inner Child Psychoanalysis, in order to uncover their deep beliefs.

3. The processes of NLP, hypnosis, or PSYCHOLOGICALSURGERY can then achieve reprogramming.

4. Each personality may require treatment, similar to other classes of The KCD. The likeliest forms are 'The Jukebox' and 'The Mountain Mule.'

5. When each personality has progressed into a more amenable belief structure, 'Combination Therapy' is required.

6. 'Combination Therapy' is a term that I have created to explain how the two personalities of one human being can be integrated. The therapy is similar to bringing together two arguing siblings from the same family. After each has worked on their own difficulties, as discussed above, they are both given a 'voice,' as if they were two separate people. They negotiate an agreement, as to how they can both co-exist fairly. By finding a middle ground, where each respects the other, then

harmony can be achieved. Inner Child Psychoanalysis and subconscious reprogramming can do this.

7. Due to the severity of this condition, medication such as lithium can be extremely useful in maintaining a stable mood.

Mrs. Fazakerly remained on her medication for many years. When she was stable, she underwent Inner Child Psychodynamic therapy. She began to understand each personality separately. Her condition improved further.

During sessions of 'Combination Therapy' she imagined the two halves of herself playing together like children. To her surprise she discovered that the 'Prince/ss' and the 'Pauper' actually liked each other. The Prince/ss could see that the Pauper was conscientious and tried to help others, whilst the Pauper discovered that the Prince/ss was fun and happy. It was as if each child recognized that what they were missing was in the other.

Mrs. Fazakerly began to meditate daily on integrating her two halves. She discovered that when she did this, her moods would regulate. She also felt safe, for the first time in years. Previously, her moods had run away with her, as one of her personalities played out. However, because 'The Prince/ss' and 'The Pauper' each had a voice, they would moderate their own behavior.

Suggested strategies to help 'THE PRINCE/SS AND THE PAUPER' class of The KCD:

1. Medication may be essential for this form of depression (as per your doctor).
2. Inner Child Psychoanalysis is advised to discover 'The Prince/ss' and 'The Pauper' separately.

3. PSYCHOLOGICALSURGERY, NLP, or hypnosis is useful for reprogramming each personality.

4. Each personality should be treated according to their class of The KCD.

5. Combination Therapy is required, in order to bring the 'Prince/ss' and the 'Pauper' together in a harmonious relationship.

6. Daily meditations, where both personalities interact with each other, are useful in maintaining a healthy relationship.

7. Different strategies created for manic and depressive phase of the condition:

    a. Have someone stop you spending large amounts when manic.

    b. Do not make major decisions when manic.

    c. Increase medication if necessary when manic.

    d. Increase exercise when low.

    e. Connect to others and do not isolate.

    f. Eat regular, healthy meals.

    g. If symptoms get worse, consult your doctor ASAP.

Chapter 10

The Empty and Overflowing Tank

(Exhaustion and Deprivation of Necessities and Toxic Stress Reaction)

This class of depression is split into two halves. They are in essence two sides of the same coin. Though at first they may seem to be the exact opposites they share many causes, symptoms and treatments.

Claire felt low every winter. She had a happy life normally but when the weather turned and the nights came in early she would want to hibernate. She lived in Edinburgh, the beautiful capital of Scotland where in winter there was little sun.

Claire worked as a civil servant and for many months went into her office in darkness and left in darkness. Her mood deteriorated as the months went by.

For Claire was exhibiting the classic symptoms of The KCD of:

9a. The Empty Tank

(Exhaustion and Deprivation of Necessities)

In Particular she had Seasonal Affective Disorder (SAD)

The common symptoms and history of this form of depression are:

1. Obvious lack in life's fundamentals such as:
    a. Nutrition (including vitamins and minerals)
    b. Water
    c. Sleep

d.   Human contact

e.   Passion

f.   Light

g.   Time for oneself.

2.   Hormone imbalance such as low thyroid levels.

3.   Low sunlight exposure (Seasonal Affective Disorder).

4.   Poor diet.

5.   Substance abuse, such as alcohol.

6.   Overworking.

Lack of sleep, poor nutrition, and lack of sunlight and time to oneself are among many internal and external factors that can cause depression. For a complete list see 'Self help' psychological options' in Chapter 20 – 'Guide to helpful processes and therapeutic substances.' The deficiency may have been caused by a negative lifestyle, such as alcohol or drug addiction, or by inadequate intake of necessities such as vitamins and minerals.

The reason for 'The Empty Tank' may be obvious and easily treated, or it may be more obscure, such as a deficiency of magnesium. Whatever the missing health factor is, it seems to lead to a decrease in serotonin levels and hence to symptoms of depression.

There have been no studies to highlight all the causes of this class of The KCD. However, I agree with Dr. Stephen Ilardi, who proclaims in his excellent book 'The Depression Cure' that five very common causes of depression are the lack of: Omega-3 fat and other nutrients, sunlight, exercise, sleep, and social connections.

Treatment of 'The Empty Tank' class of The KCD can begin with an enquiry into what may be missing in the individual's life. Compiling a list of activities, lifestyle choices and nutrition is an excellent starting point. An example of this is explained in the 'Putting it into practice' chapter at the end of the book.

A full check up from a doctor is important for all individuals suffering from depression because the cause may be hidden. Your doctor may recommend blood tests to check for hormone levels, anemia, kidney, liver, and vitamin and mineral levels.

Certain causes are more likely in different environments. For instance, those that live in low sunshine areas of the northern hemisphere may suffer from SAD. This can respond extremely well to high voltage 'Light Box Therapy' for short periods each day (approximately 10,000 lux for only 30 minutes each morning). I feel that **SAD is highly under diagnosed** when we take into account suicide rates in the more northerly countries of the northern hemisphere. I believe that Light Box Therapy should be easily available.

Individuals that live in poor urban areas may well be suffering from a nutritional malnourishment. However, this is not just a problem of the poor but is found across the board because of current Western diets and food production.

Many 'Empty Tanks' occur because of overwork and lifestyle issues, such as lack of exercise. Use of a life coach and a nutritionist can both be extremely beneficial. Other factors that maintain a happy mood include love, passion, nature, touch, and exercise. A useful tool in healing depression is for a person to write a list of what makes them happy, then to work on committing to changing their lifestyle, in order to incorporate those factors.

Claire was diagnosed with SAD and started treatment with 30 minutes of light treatment every morning. She found that after only a week her mood was reverting to normal. She continued her treatment throughout the winter.

Suggested strategies to help 'THE EMPTY TANK' class of The KCD:

1. Consider whether you are sufficient in the list below (for treatment see Chapter 20):

   a. Lack of sunlight

   b. Lack of sleep

   c. Taking depression-causing medication

   d. Substance abuse, such as alcohol or marijuana

   e. Poor nutrition

   f. Lack of relaxation

   g. Lack of love

   h. Lack of touch

   i. Lack of nature

   j. Lack of passion

   k. Lack of exercise

   l. Lack of water.

2. See a doctor for blood tests and general check up.

3. Receive professional nutritional advice.

4. Write a list of what makes you happy and commit to doing it.

5. A life coach or friend can be helpful in creating a weekly/daily routine that ensures good nutrition, sleep, exercise, and time for fun, passion, and love.

Stuart, 46, slumped down opposite me in my office. He yawned, put his head in his hands, and said, "I'm not doing well, doctor."

Stuart had become tearful and angry over the last two and a half weeks. He could not sleep properly and felt exhausted. He was working 16-hour days as a lawyer in the city. His office was very dark and his diet consisted of greasy take away food, coffee, and chocolate bars. Stuart had been divorced for 5 years and lived alone.

On a business trip to New York he had sudden chest pains and shortness of breath. He started sweating and feeling unwell. He was given oxygen and taken to hospital. They suspected a heart problem but all tests were negative apart from high blood pressure and slightly high sugar level.

He continued with anxiety attacks and feeling low, angry, and tearful.

For Stuart was exhibiting the classic symptoms of The KCD of:

9b. The Overflowing Tank
(Toxic Stress Reaction)

The common symptoms and history of this form of depression are:

1. Either a single stressful event, or more likely a culmination of events, which are too much to handle.
2. Person often becomes anxious with poor concentration and emotionally labile.
3. Anger and snappiness ensues.
4. The 'stress' of the situation often leads to the flight or fight response. This is often a chronic situation and can lead to panic attacks and the feeling of being 'wired.' This often results in:
   a. Constant state of agitation
   b. Snappiness

c. Physical symptoms such as chest pains

d. Inability to sleep

e. Weight gain

f. Helplessness

g. Fast pulse rate and palpitations.

There is an old story about a man who is so busy that he becomes depressed. He is told that a wise monk, who lives on the top of a mountain, can help him. So he rushes up this mountain in order that he can get better and get on with all his tasks. He is furious that there are no roads up the mountain and he has to walk. When he finds the monastery, he is kept waiting. This means he will be late for his next meeting. When eventually he does get to see the monk, the wise man just shrugs his shoulders and says that he cannot help him. He does, however, offer him a cup of tea. The businessman holds his cup and watches in astonishment then anger as the cup slowly fills until the liquid is at the rim. The monk continues to pour. Tea falls into the saucer and then over the edge. The man furiously throws the cup down and says, "Are you stupid, don't you know when the cup is full?"

The monk replies, "I do, but do you?"

We are not designed to be continually stressed; instead we need to be calm so that if anything life threatening occurs we can react. This reaction is called the 'flight or fight' response and is for emergencies only; when we are about to be attacked. When it turns on it causes our adrenalin and cortisol levels to rise. This in turn causes rapid heart rate, decrease in blood for digestion, high blood pressure, a raise in glucose levels, and sweating. Short term, this is a perfect response. However, if left long term it can cause exhaustion and ill health such as high blood pressure, diabetes, strokes, and heart attacks.

Treatment of 'The Overflowing Tank.' The key to this form of depression is simplicity. Learning to be idle. Idle is good, idle is natural and relaxation is the normal state for our minds and bodies. Yes, modern life is difficult but the overflowing tank will eventually lead to poor physical and mental health. So STOP. There are those things that you need to deal with and others that will need to wait. It is important to diarize relaxation time every day. It is as important as the meeting with the head of your department. A full check up is important to rule out high blood pressure and diabetes. Also, remove stimulants from your diet such as coffee, fizzy drinks, and sugary foods. Supplements such as B complex can help with adrenal glands, which have been overworking and producing high levels of cortisol and adrenalin.

Stuart was pleased to discover that all his blood test results were normal. His raised glucose was probably caused by the stress reaction and reverted to normal after a prolonged rest.

He agreed that he needed sleep, a better diet, and more sunlight. Though he had a week to go before a big deadline, he spent one day sleeping, eating healthily, and walking outdoors in the sunlight.

He learned to meditate and would spend at least half an hour a day with all phones and electrical equipment off.

Stuart visited a nutritionist. He reduced his caffeine and alcohol intake, and began eating more fruits and vegetables. Over the coming months he began to feel happier and fitter. His weight dropped. He began to cycle to work and to take his lunch in the park.

Being in a much better place, Stuart was open to other things in his life. So much so that he noticed a beautiful lady having lunch near him in the park on many occasions. He plucked up the courage and they have now been dating for 6 months.

Suggested strategies to help 'THE OVERFLOWING TANK' class of The KCD:

1. Forgive yourself for needing help.
2. Take a break.
3. Monitor your breathing – is it fast? Slow it down. The best way of doing this is to breath in for 3 seconds, hold for 3 seconds and breathe out for 3 seconds.
4. Have relaxation time in your day; every day:
    a. Walking
    b. Meditation
    c. Yoga
    d. Laughing with friends
    e. Reading.
5. Have regular breaks away from work.
6. Allow yourself to be completely idle.
7. Have a priority list and deal with the issues that you are most concerned about.
8. Medication such as benzodiazepines and beta-blockers can be useful but can lead to addictions and have side effects.
9. Cut out all stimulants such as coffee, fizzy drinks, and sugary food.
10. Exercise can help burn up that stress like feeling.
11. If ongoing symptoms, you may need a life coach, counselor or CBT to work on why you are getting so stressed and how to budget your time as listed above.

Chapter 11

Medical

(Associated Medical Illness)

John, 55, was the head of a small accountancy firm in London. He was normally very upbeat. However, over the last 3 months he had become extremely anxious and tearful. He felt scared, as if something serious needed to be addressed. So nervous, in fact, that he had reduced his eating and subsequently lost 10 pounds of weight. Yet, nothing in his life was unusual. He was doing well at work and his family life was extremely harmonious.

John could not understand his 'depression.' He had never felt like this before. His sleeping pattern became irregular and he began to feel guilty about his relationship with his now deceased father.

There was no obvious psychological cause for this. I was, however, concerned about his weight loss. On further discussion, John revealed that he had some blood in his motions a few months ago.

Following medical investigations, a diagnosis of early bowel cancer was made.

For John was exhibiting one manifestation of the classic symptoms of The KCD class of:

10. Medical

(Associated Medical Illness)

The 'Medical' class of The KCD is broadly split into two sub-types. These are anxiety and depressive symptoms that:

1. Arise as a warning system that there is an undiagnosed illness that requires attention.
2. Occur in tandem with an already diagnosed illness or use of medication.

The common symptoms and history of this entire class of depression are:

1. Feeling that something is wrong and this is an unusual feeling for that person.
2. The presence of physical symptoms, such as weight loss, shortness of breath, or undue tiredness.
3. Starting new medications such as steroids or blood pressure pills, which may cause depression.
4. Having a diagnosed major illness or hormone imbalance.

Serious illness can present with an underlying anxiety or depressed state. It may be the body's way of warning the individual that action is needed quickly. There may well be associated physical symptoms, which can include weight changes (especially weight loss), loss of appetite, shortness of breath, overtiredness, chest pains, unresolved cough, bowel or bladder symptoms, and undiagnosed pains.

Alternatively, the depression may be caused by an already diagnosed illness. Those that are particularly associated with a depressed state are hypothyroidism, anemia, diabetes, alcohol disease, and severe lung and heart disease. Depression rates for cancer patients can be as high as 50%. A number of medications can also have associations with depression, such as steroids, blood pressure tablets, and immunosuppressant drugs.

Treatment for the 'Medical' class of The KCD is both physical and psychological. Firstly, a doctor needs to be involved as soon as either an unexplained physical symptom occurs, or for depression that has health concerns attached to it. I have found that human beings have an innate ability to 'know' when there is a serious medical condition. Therefore, anxiety and/or depression can act as an early warning system, even if there are no physical symptoms.

Even when a disease is diagnosed, depression is common. This may be because other classes of The KCD are activated. However, it may be because ill individuals create visions of their future in pain, or mutilated. It is those visions and fears that can cause the depression.

It is therefore very important for people suffering from a severe illness to create a positive mindset, in order for him or her to heal, and to maintain a good mental state. A healthy and inspiring future needs to be created in the subconscious. NLP, hypnosis, or PSYCHOLOGICALSURGERY can help achieve this – as can vision boards, mantras, and meditations.

There are understandable fears and deep-seated beliefs in severe illnesses. In particular, individuals often consider that this 'should not' be happening, or that they are being punished for bad behavior. These thoughts can hinder healing and can cause depression. Therefore, expressing then releasing fears and 'shoulds' is important to enable good mental health. This will facilitate in an individual taking responsibility for getting better and avoiding blame or guilt. CBT, use of counselors, and writing 'should lists' can all be useful for this.

There is a theory, which I support, that disease may also be the result of unresolved psychological issues. Therefore, by working through these issues, the disease may abate. I recommend the use of a counselor or a specialist in health psychology. There are a number of excellent websites and books on the matter. These include Louise Hay's book and movie 'You can Heal your Life,' and Richard Moat's website www.moativationalmedicine.com

'The Empty Tank' form of depression can often coexist with this class of The KCD. Changes in hormones, medications, and lack of essentials such as vitamins and minerals may well play their part in a patient's mood. Therefore, full examination and testing by a doctor is very important.

It is also important to maintain as normal a life as possible during a prolonged illness. Sunlight, exercise, passion, love, and fun must not be ignored.

Use of medication such as SSRIs may well be indicated in this class of The KCD.

John was surprised that as soon as he was informed of his bowel cancer diagnosis, his anxiety and depression actually abated. He suddenly could sleep and eat again, even though he was scheduled for surgery.

It was confirmed that his cancer was at a very early stage. Because of this, he did not require any chemotherapy and made a full recovery.

His anxiety and depression had acted as a warning system for his illness. It had saved his life.

Suggested strategies to help the 'MEDICAL' class of The KCD:

1.   If there are physical symptoms, consult your doctor.
2.   If there are NO physical symptoms, consult your doctor.
3.   Have a full physical examination and investigations as required.
4.   Listen to your body; if you feel something is wrong, you could be right.
5.   For existing illnesses, be nice to yourself.

6. Write a 'should list' and work through it as per 'The Mountain Mule.'

7. Create a future that inspires you.

8. Have this positive future subconsciously programmed via NLP, hypnosis, and PSYCHOLOGICALSURGERY.

9. A mindset of a positive future can be maintained by use of vision boards, mantras, and meditations.

10. Medication use for those where depression has become severe.

11. Ensure excellent nutrition.

12. Consider looking at psychological causes of illness with help of counselor or CBT.

Chapter 12

Which is Your Class of Depression?

Having read the 10 distinct groups of The KCD, it is time to consider which are the classes that are relevant to you. Even those of you that do not suffer from depression may have some personality traits that fit into one of the groups.

You can either subjectively score yourself out of 10 or use the questionnaire at the front of this book. In this way, you can then pinpoint your likely class of The KCD. For some individuals more than one group may be relevant. The most severe class is best treated first. This will become clearer when you are encouraged to create your own action plan at the end of the book.

During sample testing, most people had one or two predominant classes of The KCD. However, a few individuals had a small degree of many classes. All concerned were able to create helpful action plans, which initially focused on changes relating to the most severe depressive factors. For those people whose mood was good, the information was useful in 'fine tuning' their lives, in order to feel more fulfilled.

Another issue that surfaced was that some depressed individuals noticed that one or more of their classes of The KCD were either remnants from the past or improving. This is important because if a person's current plans are working, then it may be best to continue with them. That is why it is useful to note whether the symptoms are getting better, worse, or staying the same.

From the earlier questionnaire or from your subjective marking, you may wish to fill in the table below. Mark out of 10, your score for each class of depression. Also mark down if your symptoms are getting better, worse or staying the same.

Class of the KCD	Your Score out of 10	Direction of Symptoms
1. The Mountain Mule		Better / Worse / Same
2. The Jukebox		Better / Worse / Same
3. The Stuck Trapeze		Better / Worse / Same
4. Loss Reaction		Better / Worse / Same
5. The Dynamite		Better / Worse / Same
6. Naturally Deficient		Better / Worse / Same
7. The Gravy Train		Better / Worse / Same
8. The Princess and the Pauper		Better / Worse / Same
9. The Empty and Overflowing Tank		Better / Worse / Same
10. Medical		Better / Worse / Same

In the coming chapters we will be looking at how to grade the severity of an individual's depression, which, combined with this chapter's work, will help in creating a highly personal action plan.

From the above table, you may wish to answer the following questions.
What is the predominate form of depression that you are suffering from?
Are there other forms of depression present? (Results greater than 5)
Is each class getting better, worse, or staying the same?
What form of therapy or treatment does this suggest?
What daily processes could I start to do? (For example: a 'should' list or mantras)
What investigations may be required?
What changes in lifestyle would benefit my moods?

In answering this you may wish to consider:	
How much time do I sleep?	
How much exercise do I do/ week?	
How much water do I drink?	
How many fruits/ vegetables or seeds do I consume/ day?	
Do I take multivitamins or omega 3 supplements?	
How much alcohol and caffeine do I consume weekly?	
How many sunlight hours do I have/day?	
How much time is spent on 'fun' activities per week?	
How much time is spent connecting to others socially?	
How much time do I spend in nature/ week?	
How much time do I spend meditating or deeply relaxing?	

A trusted family member or friend is often very helpful in discussing your findings with. You may feel like tackling this on your own, but the best results of treatment come when there is support. It is also vital that if you think that you have depression, that you involve your doctor or medical health practitioner in your treatment.

Name of:	
Professional	
Family / Friend	
That you will consult with, for help in your condition.	

Congratulations, you have taken a giant leap in the right direction. In recognizing the problem, you have begun to heal from it. As you continue to put steps in place, in order to overcome your depression, you will move towards happiness. When a person is on the right path, however tough it may be, there is always hope pulling them forward. Next we will look at how to grade the severity of your depression and contingency plans in overcoming a low mood.

PART 2

SEVERITY GRADING AND MOOD

MONITORING OF THE KCD

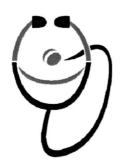

Chapter 13

Grading Your Mood

The KCD Severity Ratings

Grading the severity of an individual's condition is extremely important in overcoming depression. This is because:

1. It facilitates the individual to be the observer of their moods. This can lift them above their depressed feelings, even if this is momentary.

2. By monitoring average daily or weekly moods, an individual can assess how their depressive symptoms are progressing.

3. At certain levels of mood, preplanned interventional actions can be set into motion.

In creating this severity rating I have chosen to make the happiest mood correspond to enlightenment, at a level of 10, the lowest mood being that of catatonia (complete inability to function), at a score of 1.

I have chosen 'enlightenment' as the pinnacle of the severity ratings, because I believe that all human beings' ultimate aim is to reach this level. This aspiration combines total physical, psychological and spiritual fulfillment. Therefore, if we do not reach this level of self-actualization, then to some degree we are depressed, though this level of dysfunction may be far from a clinical illness. This way of calibrating the condition brings a number of issues to the fore:

1. Virtually every human being is suffering from some degree of 'depression.'

2. 'Clinical depression' is a line in the sand that the medical profession has drawn in deciding whom to treat.

3. Depression is a normal human state.

4. All individuals can benefit from the help this book may give.

5. The full aim of 'curing' depression is not only to function well in the world, but also to grow beyond the happiness we have known before.

Both enlightenment and catatonia are very rare. Most individuals, even with a clinical depression, will fluctuate between levels of 3 and 7 on The KCD mood severity ratings.

The KCD Questionnaire to grade your mood

Below are five main groups of questions, each of which has answers that are marked from 0 to 2. When all are totaled it can give a maximum score of 10. This corresponds to an incredible and enlightened state of mind. A score of 0–2 suggests severe depression, 3–4 moderate depression, and 5–6 a mild depression. Most individuals will score between 3 and 7.

This questionnaire can be used daily, and its uses are further highlighted in the coming chapters: Chapter 14 – 'Monitoring your mood and creating contingency policies'; Chapter 22 – 'Your daily plan.' For those who wish a deeper understanding of the scoring system, greater in depth mood tables and explanations follow after this questionnaire. Otherwise, you may wish to skip the rest of this chapter.

Are Your Thoughts	Points Score	Your Points
Mainly negative?	0	
Slightly more negative than positive?	½	
Slightly more positive than negative?	1	
Very positive?	1½	
Blissful?	2	

Are Your Thoughts	Points Score	Your Points
Mainly about fixing the past?	0	
Slightly more about the past than the future?	½	
Slightly more about the future than the past?	1	
The future being positive?	1½	
About the present?	2	

Do You Feel You Have	Points Score	Your Points
No control over your life?	0	
Slight control over your life?	½	
Good control over your life?	1	
Great deal of control, but can give some control away?	1½	
No need for control because you feel connected to others and the universe?	2	

Do you have any physical symptoms that may be caused by or causing your depression?*	Points Score	Your Points
Severe physical symptoms?	0	
Moderate physical symptoms?	½	
Slightly physical symptoms?	1	
No symptoms at all?	1½	
No, feel in fantastic physical shape?	2	

Are Your Emotions	Points Score	Your Points
Severely negative including worthlessness, guilt, anger, hopelessness, or suicidal?	0	
Moderately negative, including worthlessness, guilt, hopelessness, or anger?	½	
Very slight negative emotions, reasonably positive ones?	1	
Mainly all positive?	1½	
Fully in your control, therefore they can be switched from negative to positive easily? You remain in a healthy happy emotional state?	2	

Today's Score - Total all the above 5 Tables' points that you have scored.	Your Points
Total	/10

*These physical symptoms may include pain, being over or under weight or physically unfit, or personal specific symptoms that occur when you are depressed, such as headaches, rashes, stomach aches, or diarrhea. Alternatively, physical symptoms can include those that are related to a severe illness, such as heart disease or cancer.

An interesting use of the above questionnaire is also in predicting how your mood would be if you changed your behavior. For instance, if your score is 3 and you are very docile and overweight, what would happen to your score if you went to the gym every day? Within 6 weeks you may add between one and two points to your mood ratings. The same may apply by going to therapy, in order to relieve emotional symptoms or to change your thought patterns.

A number of patients have reflected that when they retrospectively graded themselves for previous episodes of depression, they realized that certain behavior patterns saved them from going into an abyss. Common among them included having close friends, seeing a therapist, budgeting their time and money, and working out.

Following is a more in-depth look at how and why The KCD Severity Rating system works. This information is not necessary for simply filling in the above questionnaire.

The KCD Severity Ratings

The main determinants of a depressed or happy mood in The KCD Severity Rating are:

1. State of mind and focus.
2. Belief in our own thoughts.
3. Level of control of our lives.
4. Physical/psychological symptoms.

These components are rated in the four tables below. You may wish to mark yourself as you study them, or alternatively, you can create your own scoring system. You can use any factors that you feel define the level of your mood, though changes in physical and psychological symptoms are the commonest determinants. The most important consideration is that you can have a system whereby you can accurately measure your mood daily. There is an empty table to facilitate this at the end of this chapter.

1. State of mind and focus:

Is an individual somewhere in their thoughts or completely present? If they are in their thought patterns, are they positive or negative? Are their thoughts directed at fixing the past* or are they focused more on the present and future?

*Fixing the past is the process whereby an individual imagines, or bargains with the world, that what has already happened will change. This will then alter their current situation or their projected future. This of course is impossible; the problem remains, and that person will keep in the past, rather than the present and future.

Happier moods have positive thoughts, or they are present to the moment. An example of this fully present mood is in the sports world. The athlete is said to be 'in the zone' – so focused on what they are doing that time seems to slow, and all their senses are heightened. As mood decreases, then thoughts increase. At the higher levels, the thoughts are more about the present. A middle range mood is associated with focus on the future, but this feeling decreases if the future vision is negative. At the lower end of the mood spectrum, more focus is placed on thinking about the past. Worse still is when an individual attempts to mentally 'fix' the past, as if this mental exercise will change their current reality.

2. Level of control of our lives:

People who believe they have no control over their lives are likelier to have a lower mood. As perceived control increases, mood tends to increase. Paradoxically, at the higher end of the mood spectrum, as people become more enlightened, their 'need' to be in control reduces. They voluntarily surrender their need of control to others, or to what they believe is a higher power.

3. Belief in our own thoughts:

Does an individual believe in his or her own thoughts being the only truth? If they do, then they are at the mercy of preprogrammed, often negative, ways of thinking. This person is likely to have a low mood.

As people question their own thoughts, their positive disposition tends to increase. As enlightenment follows, they create their own thought processes that are likely to result in a happy mood.

At both ends of the spectrum, there is often little true thinking. When extremely low, an individual's thoughts become so thick and dark that they stop the brain from working logically. Enlightened people can transcend their thoughts, in order to be fully present.

4. Physical/ psychological symptoms:

There are both physical and psychological symptoms of an individual's mood. The lower the mood, the likelier negative emotions are to be present. These include anger, guilt, worthlessness, and loneliness. They often result in an increase in crying, and ultimately in a false feeling that it is 'better to be dead.' Hence suicide ideation and actions can increase with a decreased mood.*

At the lower end of the spectrum, an individual feels completely disconnected from the world and their surroundings; whereas the opposite is true at the higher end. Fear, which results in forms of anxiety, is not present to those who are fully present, and can increase as their mood drops. A physical symptom, such as abdominal pain, a rash, headaches, and general aches and pains, also increases with a decreasing mood.

The exception to an improvement of symptoms with a lighter mood is that of the 'Prince/ss and the Pauper' class of The KCD. At the more 'positive end' of the mood spectrum, manic symptoms and a disconnectedness from the world occurs. This is because the 'prince/ss's addictive mind patterns are taking over.

*I believe that suicide attempts are not entirely proportional to a negative mood. In fact, I find that a number of cases are due to mental programs that exist in the subconscious. Some suicide attempts occur as a patient's mood improves.

1. State of mind and focus		
Level of happiness	*State of mind*	*Focus*
10	Not thinking. Just being.	Fully present
9	Blissful, grateful	Virtually fully present
8	Happy, grateful, confident of good future	Present and future
7	Happy, few concerns re future, optimistic. Past thoughts insignificant and often positive.	Present, more future slight past
6	Content, concerns re future and past generally positive.	Past, future similar
5	Concerns and worries moderate re future. Still 'fixing past'.	Fixing past and future, state of no change
4	Most time spent on fixing past and viewing negative future.	Past, and frightened of future
3	Living in past, cannot face future	Past predominates and needs fixing
2	Cannot face future or past	World turning too black to think straight.
1	Totally shut down	Totally black state of mind.

2. Level of control of our lives, and 3. Belief in our own thoughts:		
Level of happiness	*State of mind*	*Focus*
10	Nil required, full trust in universe (past and future do not exist).	Totally surrenders to the universe, still takes all appropriate actions.
9	Present most of the time.	Surrenders almost completely to the universe, still takes all appropriate actions.
8	Excellent control of staying present and creating future.	Can control thought process, knowing it is a tool and not the truth.
7	Good control of present and future mindsets and easily can switch out of past memories.	Knows that the answer may be inside them or outside. Happy to share decisions
6	Increasing control over past negative memories, and can control having more positive memories of past. Increased control of positive future thoughts, and ability to become 'present'.	Feels own thoughts maybe right, but will get second opinions and help.
5	Feels has some control over reducing negative past emotions, and can start to create positive future thoughts.	Feels own thoughts maybe right, but will get second opinions and help if really pushed.
4	Little control over present feelings, future events and past. Time spent thinking about past and future similar. But thoughts more negative than positive.	Their thoughts are sinking them and feel real. They are willing to ask for help.
3	Virtually no control over feelings, the future not existing and no control over past. Mainly thinking about negative past.	Their thoughts are sinking them deeper and feel real. They are becoming childlike or isolates, and will not get any help.
2	No control of being in the negative mind patterns of the past all the time.	What they think is true; there is nothing anyone can do about it. Too low to ask for help. It feels like there is no point anyway.
1	No control of being in hell (past, present and future do not exist).	Too black to think anything.

3. Physical/ psychological symptoms:

Level of happiness	Normal	For 'The Prince/ss and the Pauper' only
10	Fully alive, pulsating beautiful energy. Totally connected to world.	Feels like they own the world; they are divine.
9	Fully alive, pulsating beautiful energy. In love with the world.	Feel that they could save the world and have no responsibility for actions. They spend and play excessively.
8	Laughing and smiling predominate. Feeling great most of the time.	Laughing and smiling predominate. Feeling great most of the time.
7	Excited for life and happy.	Excited for life and happy.
6	Stable, mild anxieties, life seems balanced. Slight physical symptoms such as abdominal pain or headaches may occur.	Stable, mild anxieties, life seems balanced. Slight physical symptoms such as abdominal pain or headaches may occur.
5	Just stable, mild to moderate anxieties, concerns that things may get worse, moderate concentration. Moderate physical symptoms such as abdominal pain or headaches may occur.	Just stable, mild to moderate anxieties, concerns that things may get worse, moderate concentration. Moderate physical symptoms such as abdominal pain or headaches may occur.
4	Has a feeling of getting out of control, increasing mild to moderate anger, guilt and worthlessness. Seeking love from others. Moderate to severe physical symptoms such as abdominal pain or headaches may occur.	Has a feeling of getting out of control, increasing mild to moderate anger, guilt and worthlessness. Seeking love from others. Moderate to severe physical symptoms such as abdominal pain or headaches may occur.
3	Life is out of control, high anger, guilt and worthlessness, crying and hiding from people. Severe physical symptoms such as abdominal pain or headaches occur. Moderate Suicidal ideas.	Life is out of control, high anger, guilt and worthlessness, crying and hiding from people. Severe physical symptoms such as abdominal pain or headaches occur. Moderate Suicidal ideas.
2	Wild fluctuations of anger, guilt and worthlessness. Uncontrolled crying, do not want to live, feeling of no way out. Severe physical symptoms such as abdominal pain or headaches occur. Severe Suicidal ideas.	Wild fluctuations of anger, guilt and worthlessness. Uncontrolled crying, do not want to live, feeling of no way out. Severe physical symptoms such as abdominal pain or headaches occur. Severe Suicidal ideas.
1	So black not aware of extreme emotions or physical pains.	So black not aware of extreme emotions or physical pains.

Your own scoring system

You may choose to create your own scoring system based on your specific symptoms, which correlates with a particular level of your mood. There is a blank table below that you may wish to fill in.

In creating your own scoring system, you may wish to consider patterns in your own life. For instance, does your low mood correlate with lack of exercise, changes in diet, tiredness, or stress in your life? What physical symptoms do you tend to get at different levels of your mood? These can include headaches, abdominal pains, rashes, bowel or bladder frequency, or aches and pains. Other symptoms that may be relevant include your eating habits and compulsions, your weight, or the clothes you tend to wear. Some people find changes in spending money, ability to concentrate, and the amount of socializing alter with level of mood.

In most cases, knowing your symptoms at either end of the spectrum is unlikely. So I suggest you fill in the levels of 5 and 6 first and expand from there as you can.

Level of happiness	State of mind	Thoughts and symptoms
10		
9		
8		
7		
6		
5		
4		
3		
2		
1		

Chapter 14

Monitoring Your Mood and Creating Contingency Policies

Whether you use The KCD grading system or your own, monitoring your mood daily will give you more control of your life. The information gleaned can lead to a greater understanding of your depression. It may shed light on the cause and the progression of your condition. This is best viewed month by month, after plotting average daily mood severities.

As shown in the table below, a monthly table of moods can be color coded for the severity of your condition. This is useful for being able to put contingency policies into place.

Level of happiness is split into four separate color regions. These sections are:

7–10–	green shading–	a happy individual.
5–6–	yellow shading–	mild depressive symptoms.
3–4–	blue shading–	moderate depressive symptoms.
1–2–	red shading–	severe depressive symptoms.

	Day of the Month																														
vel	*1*	*2*	*3*	*4*	*5*	*6*	*7*	*8*	*9*	*10*	*11*	*12*	*13*	*14*	*15*	*16*	*17*	*18*	*19*	*20*	*21*	*22*	*23*	*24*	*25*	*26*	*27*	*28*	*29*	*30*	*31*
0																															
7																															
	1	*2*	*3*	*4*	*5*	*6*	*7*	*8*	*9*	*10*	*11*	*12*	*13*	*14*	*15*	*16*	*17*	*18*	*19*	*20*	*21*	*22*	*23*	*24*	*25*	*26*	*27*	*28*	*29*	*30*	*31*

OSTER POLICY - implement in 3-7 days

ERMEDIATE POLICY - implement in 1-2 days

ISIS POLICY - immediate action

By viewing daily and weekly changes in your moods, you can quickly isolate a negative trend. Planned interventions can then be instigated if your depression reaches certain levels or remains low for some time. The deeper the depression, the quicker the intervention needs to be.

The creation of interventions is best done before a crisis occurs. This is because the deeper a depressed mood, the more difficult it is to formulate a plan. In creating these plans or policies, I suggest the following recommendations:

1. Create your plans with help of friends and family.
2. Make the plans simple.
3. Make sure all the information on the form is accurate.
4. Make three separate plans for mild, moderate, and severe episodes. These policies can be activated after varying lengths of time.
5. Choose when to implement each policy. For mild depression, you may choose to wait up to a week before taking action, whereas for severe depression you may need to implement immediately.

103

Rules to creating your policies could include the following:

1. Write this policy when you are feeling happy and can concentrate.

2. Tell all the people that may become involved in implementing your policy what may be expected of them. Make sure they agree fully. If they do not fully agree, then find another person to fill this void. Remember, everybody has the right to say 'NO.'

3. Have each policy easily accessible. This can be on your phone or computer or in a diary.

4. Have all material ready for activation of a policy, such as music, DVDs, and contact details.

5. Activate policy when you said you would.

Policies may include:

1. People to call for help.

2. Their contact details.

3. Procedures for getting out of a low mood.

4. Activities that raise the mood.

5. Photograph that can raise the mood.

6. Questioning as to why you may have become depressed this time.

'10 simple paths to happiness' examples of policies

Below are three policies that you may wish to use. They include:

1. A Booster policy for mild depressive symptoms.

2. An intermediate policy for moderate depressive symptoms.

3. Crisis policy for severe depressive symptoms.

My suggestion for **activation of these policies** is shown below.

However, apart from the crisis policy, they are merely estimates. When you create your own policies, then you can choose when they 'should' be activated.

BOOSTER POLICY –   **implement in 3–7 days**

INTERMEDIATE POLICY –   **implement in 1–2 days**

CRISIS POLICY –   **immediate action**

Contingency Policies

BOOSTER POLICY – MILD Level 5-6		
1. What is happening? Are you getting enough Sleep, Exercise, Fun, Laughter, Sunlight, Good food? Are you taking your medicines properly?	What will you do today to improve?	
2. What fears do you have about your future? Now how do you want your future to be?	What 1 action can you take today to make this happen?	
3. What do you feel that you have no control over?	Can you do something about it or accept it?	
4. Who are you going to chat with, to help you create your future and to deal with what is going on?	a. name a. number	b. name b. number
5. Arrange something fun into your diary, this can be booking a holiday or arranging to see friends.		
6. Choose a book, music or DVD, a fun activity, or something you are passionate about and do it.	My choice is:	
7. If you have a daily plan of action then revisit you daily plan – put in actions.	Monitor level if: a. The same, repeat this Policy (A) b. If worse, go to INTERMEDIATE POLICY (B)	

INTERMEDIATE POLICY – MODERATE Level 3-4		
1. What is happening? Are you getting enough: Sleep, Exercise, Fun, Laughter, Sunlight, Good food? Are you taking your medicines properly?	What will you do today to improve?	
2. What are you fearful of? LET IT OUT ON PAPER		
3. What do you need to forgive yourself or others for?		
4.What is happening in Reality?	So What?	Now What?
5.Write 5 'SHOULDS' that you are telling yourself.	1 2 3 4 5	
Repeat Mantra 10 times: I DESERVE TO BE HAPPY. I AM WORTHWHILE AND I FORGIVE OTHERS AND MYSELF FULLY FOR WHERE I AM NOW.		
6. I need to inform the agreed people or person of my current mood. They are:	a. name b. name c. name	a. number b. number c. number
7. Choose a book, music, or DVD that improves your mood, and spend time doing that.	My choice is:	
8. Make appointment with doctor or mental health practitioner. Monitor level, if	a. The same, repeat this Policy (B)	
	b. If worse, go to CRISIS POLICY (C)	
	c. If better, go to THE BOOSTER PLAN.	

CRISIS POLICY – SEVERE Level 1-2		
1. Breathe deeply and slowly for 10 breaths.		
2. Mantra – repeat to yourself 3 times *I AM LOVED AND APPRECIATED. THIS* *TOO WILL PASS. I WILL FEEL BETTER.*		
3. Put on chosen music, which is:		
4. Have you taken you normal medication, if not, then take it.		
5. Let out a huge scream or cry, if necessary.		
6. Call designated person in order NOW – all the numbers should be there. Who are you going to ask for help (doctor, therapist, friend, peer, mentor?)	a. name b. name c. name d. name e. name	a. number b. number c. number d. number e. number
7. Get urgent appointment with Doctor, psychiatric nurse or psychologist as appropriate.		
8. There needs to be someone with you at all times. *Photo of loved ones:*		

PART 3

PRACTICAL ASPECTS OF THE KCD

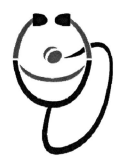

Chapter 15

The Tug of War of Life

There is a tug of war in everybody's life, between happiness and depression. On one side 'of the rope' there are behaviors that are pulling towards a person's happiness, and on the other are those that are dragging the individual towards depression. The greater the force on one side, the more likely it is to win. Below are the three aspects of behavior that will exert these forces.

1. **Actions:** It is often the actions we take that lead us to the life we want to live. Positive actions can include anything from eating healthily to taking your son to a football match. In many cases, putting in the correct actions towards happiness may feel strange or futile if the individual has been depressed for some time. However, if they continue with positive actions, they will eventually be rewarded with a positive result.

2. **Inactions:** Inaction may have as powerful an effect as action. In certain circumstances, 'doing nothing' can help in raising the mood, such as if the individual is exhausted and requires rest. However, if inaction constitutes avoiding socializing and over-thinking, then it may create a negative force. The truth of whether inactivity is pulling you towards or away from happiness is in the result. If a person feels more depressed following idle episodes, then it is likely that reducing these will help the patient.

3. **Thoughts:** Though thoughts can spontaneously enter our minds, human beings have the ability to refocus them. Individuals who remain happy and successful invariably check their thoughts, and work on altering them into positive mind patterns. This skill may have been

learnt in childhood, but can be grasped at any age. This ability of actively filtering negative thoughts and substituting positive ones is particularly important in the treatment of 'The Jukebox' class of The KCD.

There are also many external factors that can affect an individual's mood. It is the actions and thoughts taken in response to these situations that are important in winning the tug of war of life.

The ultimate tug of war of life

Whatever part of 'life' we look at, there is always a tug of war being played out. Unhealthy food pulls towards obesity, whereas exercise exerts its influence in the direction of health. Money put into a bank increases riches, spending can lead to poverty. The greatest tug of war in life is that between fear and love. Fear stops a person really living their life, whilst love does the opposite.

During many of my seminars, I have invited the audience to write down the results of their life that they are happy with and those that they are not. I get them to consider the moment they made those decisions. Were they acting out of fear or love? Invariably those decisions that turned out well were created from an aspect of love, whilst poor outcomes occurred when decisions were made out of fear.

The same principle occurs when looking at the actions, inactions, and thoughts relating to an individual's mood. Those made from a fear base often result in negative moods, whilst those from an aspect of love for life result in a positive disposition. This is extremely important in creating the behavior patterns for our futures. Choosing those actions that are from a place of love rather than fear is likely to result in a happier mood.

By choosing behaviors that increase your happiness, you get a double effect. You get the positive pull towards happiness, and the strain from the contrary attitude is no longer having an effect. In this way, a small change in demeanor can result in large alterations of mood. The tug of war of life can then be won.

A positive pull towards happiness may be the actions contained in The KCD as well as other non-specific actions that you will be encouraged to consider later in the book. However, it is important for all individuals to learn which are their positive and which are their negative behavior patterns. Then they can choose to implement and avoid activities in keeping with their aim to create a happy life. I suggest completing the tables below as a starting point to achieve this.

Behaviors pulling you towards happiness:	
1	
2	
3	
4	
5	
6	
7	
8	
9	
10	

You may also benefit from looking at events in your life, and then recalling if your decisions were from a place of fear or love of life. Decide if the results were good or bad. This may help you in making your choices in the future. This can be achieved by filling in the table opposite.

Behaviors pulling you away from happiness:	
1	
2	
3	
4	
5	
6	
7	
8	
9	
10	

You may also benefit from looking at events in your life, and then recalling if your decisions were from a place of fear or love of life. Decide if the results were good or bad. This may help you in making your choices in the future. This can be achieved by filling in the table opposite.

Event or Action	Result	Decision Made out of love of life or fear
	Good / Bad	Love / Fear
	Good / Bad	Love / Fear
	Good / Bad	Love / Fear
	Good / Bad	Love / Fear
	Good / Bad	Love / Fear
	Good / Bad	Love / Fear
	Good / Bad	Love / Fear
	Good / Bad	Love / Fear
	Good / Bad	Love / Fear
	Good / Bad	Love / Fear

The step-by-step approach:

Having created the tables above, you may wish to alter many aspects of your life all at once. However, though this can work well for some, many individuals burn out with this approach. Adjusting one or two factors first, and then integrating other changes when this feels right, is more likely to result in a lifelong positive way of being. Small changes can actually have a large effect. Also, as an individual carries out more positive actions and feels better, it becomes easier to do even more positive actions. So remember, little by little can make huge changes.

Little metamorphoses are easier to accomplish than sudden large ones. All an individual needs to do is to focus on that **one** shift until it becomes natural for them. At this point another alteration can be instigated.

This step-by-step approach can also be complemented by creating a positive vision of the future. The imagination can be used to pull the individual towards it. If, however, a person tries to work out the logical steps, they often find that the process is too complicated. They may become disheartened. Life does not work in logical steps. Highly successful people will testify that even when they planned their ventures fully, other unexpected factors came into play. What is often required in life is to take the next step, even if you cannot see the one further in front. When you have completed that one, the next will come into view.

Below is an example of how little by little can help win 'the tug of war of happiness.'

Mark was diagnosed with 'The Dynamite' class of The KCD. Over many years of keeping his emotions inside, he had become depressed. From not crying for 20 years, he started weeping every day. He also became very angry at the least provocation. At 30 years of age, he was 50 pounds over weight, living with his parents, single, and suffering from lower back pain.

Together we wrote an action plan, taking into account the behaviors that were likely to lead to his happiness. He agreed that he would take a step-by-step approach in implementing them.

This plan included:

Find a 'Journey Practitioner.'

Under go a Journey Process for treatment of 'The Dynamite.'

At the weekend go for a walk.

Write the vision of the future he wants.

Join a gym.

Have a massage or spa twice a month.

Eat healthily.

Go to 170 pounds (he was 180 pounds).

Start dating and find a partner.

Buy a property.

Go out with friends once a week.

Mark started by going for a short walk each day. He then elicited the help of his friend Claire, in order to create a vision board for his future. He began to look at this every day. By the end of the first week he had also gained the details of a 'Journey Practitioner.'

After a few weeks of walking, he decided to join a gym. At first, he just went inside, used the sauna, had a coffee and left. After a few more weeks, he began cycling on the bike for 10 minutes at a time. He persuaded Claire to join him at the gym and they both steadily increased their exercise.

Mark began to feel better and decided to alter his diet. He did this little by little. He reduced his coffee and alcohol intake and increased his fresh fruits and vegetables. The fitter he became, the healthier the foods he wished to consume.

It was many months later that he went to see a Journey Practitioner, but addressed his emotional issues over a number of sessions. He also found that by increasing his exercise, his mood improved significantly.

In six months, his weight loss was approaching 30 pounds and he had moved out from his parents' house. He began dating and found that his mood was consistently good.

Chapter 16

Tricks For Getting Out Of Depression

An indispensable skill that many happy people possess is the ability to get out of a bad mood quickly. Just because they wake up feeling low does not mean that the rest of the day has to spoil.

It is fundamental that all individuals learn ways of swiftly switching a negative to a positive mindset. For people unaccustomed to this, various techniques must seem like magic. Below are 12 of these procedures or 'tricks.' At the end of the chapter, you may wish to practice a number of them or create your own.

1. Escaping the mind

The mind is like a muscle. When it is overused, it needs to rest. Unfortunately, when people suffer from depression they can try to over-think their way out of their moods. This exhausts the brain further and can lead to more depression. It is similar to pumping heavier weights at the gym after the bicep muscles are injured.

The trick is to stop thinking and to focus energy elsewhere in the body. Going for a walk, doing something you are passionate about, such as painting or being engrossed in a great film, all qualify. However, a guided meditation is an excellent way of doing this. I have given you one of mine below but there are many available on the web and CDs.

In a safe environment lie down and close your eyes. Start to slow your breathing. Breathe in for 3 seconds, hold it for 3 seconds and blow it out for 3 seconds. Then imagine the energy in your head has a color and a shape. Is it moving? Is it changing? See the color becoming a deep red and the shape changing to be spherical. If it is spinning in

one direction, start spinning it in the other. Now imagine lifting all this
energy out of your head, like a balloon floating out of your skull. Let it
ascend above your head, up to the roof and then above the building that
you are in. Now let if fly away forever.

Place your hand on your heart and imagine that there is mass of
love and happiness. This has a color and shape. Increase the size of it,
and then make the color even more vivid. Let it fill your entire chest
and then your abdomen. Concentrate fully on this mass and the feeling
around it. Let it then fill your head. Now imagine there is an elevator
from your head down to your groin. Put all this color into the elevator
and bring it down to your throat. Let it out there and monitor what you
see and feel. Put it back in the elevator and do the same in the regions
of your heart, abdomen, and groin. Leave the energy where it feels the
most relaxed and slowly bring yourself back to consciousness. How do
you feel now?

Other excellent ways of moving your energy away from you mind
include:

a.   Deep slow breathing

b.   Yoga

c.   Sport.

2. Blowing up the balloon of unhappiness

I want you to imagine that your unhappiness is the air in a balloon.
If your 'unhappiness' rates as 6/10 then the balloon is 60% full of air.
The usual impulse is to plead with your thoughts and feelings to go
away and hence deflate the balloon. However, sometimes this results in
more air entering, or the balloon deflating a little before reacquiring air.

I want you to imagine increasing the air in the balloon. This will
mean a rise in negative thoughts and emotions. I want you to see in

your mind's eye the air increasing from 60% full to 70%. Then up to 80%, then 90%. Now you will get to 100%. So hold on. I want you to pump even more air into it. The balloon is really stretching now. It's at 110% and now 120%. Keep imagining air going into the balloon. Wait for it ......POP!

Now how do you feel?

In many cases, people feel much better. This is because emotions and thoughts can cause only so much pain. When they increase beyond this, then the mind shuts down to them in the same way a balloon goes pop. You can use this technique literally, by increasing your current thoughts and feelings, or by using this balloon meditation.

This technique may cause initial increase in anxiety; therefore I suggest that you try this with the help of a mental health practitioner. I certainly feel that you should not attempt this alone at first.

3. Become present

You cannot be present and be depressed. Really, it is impossible. For depression is a disorder of the mind and being present means that the conscious or 'thinking' mind is not thinking; it is doing. Being present means that your five senses of vision, hearing, smell, taste, and touch are unimpeded by thoughts. If you are concentrating fully on these five senses, then there is no more room for your conscious mind to think. In order to fully concentrate on your senses, all you need to do is to ask yourself what each of your senses is doing. Simply go through the questions below:

What do I see?

What do I hear?

What do I feel?

What do I taste?

What do I smell?

Continue this for at least 2 minutes:

"What do I see?

What do I hear?

What do I feel?

What do I taste?

What do I smell?

What do I see?

What do I hear?

What do I feel?

What do I taste?

What do I smell?

What do I see?

What do I hear?

What do I feel?

What do I taste?

What do I smell?"

4. Mantras

Mantras are statements that you repeat to yourself in order for them to seep into the subconscious. They are statements that reflect what you want for your life or that moment. In many cases a mantra may include a sentence that is exactly opposite to what your internal monologue is telling you. For instance, in 'The Mountain Mule' class of The KCD, individuals may have an underlying belief that 'I am not good enough.' Therefore, a mantra which begins to attack this belief would be: 'I am good enough.'

If you wake up in a bad mood you may wish to repeat a simple mantra such as 'I am happy and lucky.' This will at first feel strange and may even sound like a lie. However, after many recitals it may well become second nature.

"I am happy and lucky

I am happy and lucky

I am happy and lucky

I am happy and lucky

I am happy and lucky"

What mantra could you repeat to yourself?

....

5. Anchoring your happiness

Anchoring is a method that is used in NLP. It uses the principle of conditioning. When two senses are stimulated at the same time, they become linked. Next time one sense occurs, the other may be activated. An example would be that if your grandma always baked you apple pies, in the future, every time you smell apple pie you are reminded of your grandma. You can use any of your five senses to be anchored. Below is a simple method for anchoring relaxation and a happy mood. This procedure is best done by an NLP practitioner, though can be done alone.

You need to become relaxed and happy. So imagine the happiest you could be in your life. Everything you want is happening. All the people you like are there. Breathe slowly, and when you are feeling relaxed and happy, place the tip of your thumb and forefinger together. Now ask yourself, in this image:

"What do I see?

What do I hear?

What do I feel?

What do I taste?

What do I smell?

What do I see?

What do I hear?

What do I feel?

What do I taste?

What do I smell?

What do I see?

What do I hear?

What do I feel?

What do I taste?

What do I smell?"

Keep doing this until you feel extremely happy. Now you have a possible anchor. Next time you are feeling sad, press your fingers together as before, and breathe slowly. The mind will take you back to that happy emotional state.

What memory or thought can you use as an anchor?

....

6. Think of happy memories even if they made up

Immerse yourself in happy memories of your past. Make them even happier than you recall. You can even make up happy experiences. It's the feeling of happiness that is important.

What happy memories do you have?

....

7. Shock your system awake

People who are depressed are not fully awake. Therefore you can be shocked into 'waking up.' Anything that clicks an individual into consciousness will work. One option is to have a friend or partner clap their hands and shout 'IT'S TIME TO WAKE UP!' Another is getting into a very cold shower for 2 minutes.

What can you do to shock the system awake?

....

8. Laugh for no reason

It is very hard to stay depressed when laughing. So if you are in a socially acceptable place, make yourself laugh, even if it feels absolutely crazy to do so. Keep doing it until your mood lifts and laughing feels natural for you. You may wish to do it with others or alone.

What makes you laugh?

……………….......……………………………………..

9. Singing and music

I have found that singing and music are amongst the quickest ways of changing a mood. You may have a particular song that works best for you. You may accompany a recorded version of a song or just 'belt' one out in the shower. The more heart and soul you put into it, the quicker your mood will alter. Playing musical instruments may create the same positive result.

What music makes you feel good?

……………………………………………………....

10. Sudden burst of exercise and dancing

A quick burst of exercise is another excellent way of getting out of a depressed mood. Five minutes of either fast running, doing weights, press-ups, or sit-ups can switch a mood around. Dancing is another excellent way of getting into a positive state. It is when you least feel like doing it that the exercise is most needed.

What dancing or exercise can you do?

....

11. Doing the opposite to what your feelings are telling you

When depression occurs, it often leaves an individual feeling isolated, hard done by, and unsupported. However, by putting in actions which are diametrically opposed to the underlying thoughts, those thoughts can be challenged. Suggested actions are:

1. Write a list of 10 things you are grateful for.
2. Speak to another individual, but focus on helping them.
3. Do a charitable act.
4. If feeling poor, give some money to charity; even if it is one penny.

What actions could you take?

....

12. Blow your thoughts apart – 'The Three Whats'*

Many negative thoughts that individuals have either never come to fruition or turn out to be false. These thoughts, however, lead to negative emotions and depressive symptoms. Challenging these thoughts directly can help switch around your emotional state. There are a number of ways to do this. One is by CBT and another is using the four questions of Byron Katie's 'The Work,' which is further discussed in Chapter 20.

The simplest way to challenge thoughts, though, is by a three-line process called **'The Three Whats.'** These three questions take a thought process from the problem into the solution. It can remove drama, opinions, and blame. 'The Three Whats' are:

WHAT is really happening in reality?

*So **WHAT?***

*Now **WHAT?***

You can apply any scenario to 'The Three Whats.'

Which scenario could you choose to work on?

....

WHAT is really happening in reality?

....

So **WHAT?**

Now **WHAT?**

....

*I discovered 'The Three Whats' whilst chatting with a group of people around a campsite fire in Hawaii. I am unaware of their origin.

Chapter 17

Responsibility versus Shame

Being fully responsible for your own life and mood is the only way to be fully free of depressive symptoms. This is because it puts an individual in charge of their life, and avoids a victim state of mind. However, many people do not wish to take on responsibility for a number of reasons, including:

1. **Responsibility and shame**: People often feel that they could not deal with all the **shame,** and hence the negativity that comes with being **responsible** for the 'bad' stuff in their lives.

2. **Life is out of their control**: How can you take responsibility for yourself, when so many influential factors are external?

3. **We do not choose who we are**: Individuals argue that they did not 'choose' their genetic code, parents, race, social class, and childhood influences.

1. Responsibilities and shame

The misconceptions, which the word itself conveys, may well explain the reluctance in people accepting responsibility. This is in part caused by the false belief that blame and shame are naturally associated with it. This is clarified by the dictionary descriptions below.

'*Responsibility* is the obligation to carry forward an assigned task to a successful conclusion. With responsibility goes authority to direct and take the necessary action to ensure success'* *From 'Wikipedia'

'*To **blame*** is to hold another person or group responsible for perceived faults; real, imagined, or merely invented for pejorative purposes. Blame is an act of censure, reproach, and often outright* *condemnation. Blame is used to place responsibility and accountability for faults on the blamed person or group.'* *From 'Wikipedia'

*'**Shame** – a painful feeling of humiliation or distress caused by the consciousness of wrong or foolish behavior* – 'shame,' Oxford Dictionaries, April 2010 –

http://oxforddictionaries.com/definition/english/shame

A **responsible** person takes authority over his or her life and makes choices accordingly. It is forward thinking, and therefore works on the **solution**. No opinion needs to happen in the action taken from a purely responsible individual.

Blame is an opinion that someone or something is at fault, including him or herself, which is termed '**guilt**.' When this blame causes a sense of humiliation and paints that individual as either incompetent or bad, it becomes **shame**. It keeps the individual's focus on the **problem** and the past. It can be particularly prevalent in those forms of depression which tend to avoid life progression. This includes 'The Jukebox,' 'The Stuck Trapeze,' and 'The Gravy Train' classes of The KCD. 'The Mountain Mule' tends to exhibit guilt.

I believe that shame will keep a person in a depressed state, whereas responsibility will free them. It is therefore fundamental to divorce the terms 'responsibility' and 'shame' to their original meanings. Individuals can take responsibility for creating a solution and allow the problem and blame to subside.

Shaming someone can be like shouting at a five year old child for getting a math sum wrong. Just because outcomes in life do not turn out how you wanted does not mean that people were malicious or neglectful. In many cases people were just doing the best they could. The problem is that if you remain in a state of shame, you will increase feelings of resentment and anger, and inhibit solution finding and life progression. These will increase the symptoms of depression. This is encapsulated in the anonymous quote 'Not forgiving someone is like drinking poison and expecting the other person to die.'

2. Life is out of their control

There are many external factors that seem to affect a person's life that are out of an individual's control. However, there is a responsibility for accepting what is, and making the most of a situation. There are always choices that can be made at any moment, even if the choice is to maintain a happy mood, or to learn a lesson from what is happening. In 'Man's Search for Meaning' Viktor Frankl describes his time in a Nazi concentration camp, where there was a myriad of behaviors that his fellow inmates exhibited. Some became selfish and stole food, whilst others tried to remain cheerful and gave some of their rations to others, despite the inhumane conditions.

This story also suggests that we all need to take responsibility for our own thoughts. Negative thoughts come into every person's head, often uninvited, but it is our choice to believe and continue focusing on them. We also cannot blame others for our own feelings. Nobody opens up an individual's skull, finds the part of the brain that switches on anger or depression, and presses it. Responsibility gives a person more personal power for his or her own thoughts and feelings. They can react with greater integrity to a situation.

An example of this comes in the all too common arena of abusive relationships. In many cases, the victim stays in a dangerous relationship for far too long. They often feel low, powerless, and shame the other for their depression and upset. These emotions can then result in that person's inertia. If they were able to take responsibility for the situation, they would take action. This may include involving police, leaving the relationship, and looking at why they chose that relationship in the first place.

3. We do not choose who we are

The other common reasons that individuals refuse to take responsibility for their lives are that they did not choose many of the factors of their childhoods. They were not privy to the decisions of their place of birth, parents, siblings, school, religion, sex, or physical attributes. Every individual is born with a different life to live. Each is dealt a different hand. It is the playing of that hand that is important. People from poor backgrounds can become rich. One religion can be switched for another. Individuals can create a life completely analogous to the beliefs of their parents.

The question I ask many patients is, "At what age are you going to stop blaming (and often shaming) your parents and live your life?" Many are still holding onto the negativity of their childhood experiences into their dotage.

In some of my seminars, I ask the attendees to pretend that all their woes are in a bag at the back of the room. When they leave they can pick up their own or another's. They invariably pick up their own baggage. This is because they know what it is, and it feels that it belongs to them. They do not want to be working through someone else's 'stuff.'

I therefore feel it is time for all adults to stop blaming the past for where they are, and to take responsibility for creating the present and future.

In conclusion, when an individual takes responsibility and avoids any form of shame for their life and thoughts, their mind often clears.

This is because drama, opinions, emotions, and story disappear. They can then choose the plan of action and way of thinking that they consider is their best option. They will not know what will happen in the future but can alter their plans accordingly, to the results they are getting in their life.

For a person to forgive others is important in moving on with that person's life. This can be purely for their own mental health, for not doing this can cause anger, resentment, and ultimately disease.

For issues that an individual feels are their fault, I suggest seeking forgiveness from others and themselves. Apologize, and try to make up to the individuals affected. If others will not forgive, despite adequate recompense, then it is probably time to move on.

Chapter 18

Boundaries

When a person is unable to maintain healthy boundaries, it can lead to stress, uncertainty and negative emotions. This can be both a symptom and a cause of depression. In fact, individual classes of The KCD have different boundary issues.

The main 'boundaries' which humans need to maintain are: physical, emotional, financial, spiritual, sexual, and social.

Boundary setting begins in early childhood when an infant learns to say 'NO.' Although boundary maintenance changes with age, much of the boundary settings of an adult are as a result of their early experiences. All boundary issues lead to isolation and difficulties in relating to the self and others.

If an individual's experience of growing up was unsafe, then it is likely that very tight boundaries were created. This means that close relationships will be difficult. These tight boundaries can often be part of 'The Jukebox' and 'The Gravy Train' classes of The KCD.

If a person's childhood experience was that they had to take on a parent's role and look after others, then boundary settings may be very lax. They are unable to refuse in helping others. This can occur if one or both parents were unable to fulfill their family responsibilities. This person is then taken advantage of by others and eventually becomes sick and exhausted. This is often the case in 'The Mountain Mule' class of The KCD.

A simplified way of looking at an individual's boundary is their ability either to hear a 'YES' or a 'NO' and to ask for a 'YES' or a 'NO' from others.

The four boundary issues

This 'YES/ NO' way of looking at boundaries is explained excellently by Dr. Henry Cloud and Dr. John Townsend in their book entitled 'Boundaries....' They describe boundary issues in the four extremes of:

1. Those that cannot say 'No,' which they call 'The compliant.'
2. Those that cannot hear 'No,' which they call 'The controller.'
3. Those that cannot say 'Yes,' which they call 'The non-responsive.'
4. Those that cannot hear 'Yes,' which they call 'The avoidant.'*

*Taken from 'Boundaries: When to say yes when to say no, to take control of your life' by Dr. Henry Cloud and Dr. John Townsend. Copyright © 1992 by Dr. Henry Cloud and Dr. John Townsend. Use by permission of Zondervan. www.zondervan.com

1. The compliant: 'Can't say NO'

The compliant feels that they 'should' help others, beyond their remit and 'cannot' say 'NO.' They are often resentful that they are doing things that they do not want to, but have an inner belief that this is their job. If they do say 'NO,' they are invariably filled with guilt. They are often exhausted and run into the ground. This state of affairs was likely set in motion by having increased responsibility as a child, such as looking after a younger sibling. This form of boundary problem is characteristic of 'The Mountain Mule.'

When a compliant starts to learn to say 'NO,' others around them may find it difficult to accept these new boundaries, and perhaps increase forms of anger or manipulation to get them to say 'YES.' This is particularly relevant if the relationship is between a compliant and a controller. It may be difficult for the compliant to maintain a reasonable boundary and to say 'NO' because at first they often feel guilty for doing so. However, with practice and support, a compliant can learn to say 'NO' and to normalize their boundary position.

2. The controller: 'Can't hear NO'

Like a petulant child, the controller cannot hear a 'NO' from others. For this response is deemed unfair and unacceptable. The controller will command with either an aggressive or manipulative approach. They can switch from being charming to bossy, or to playing the victim, depending on what appears to work best.

The underlying internal monologue of a controller can often be that nobody loves them, or that they are unworthy. It may well be the result of an abusive upbringing, or an inability to grow up and see other people's point of view. The controller is prevalent in 'The Jukebox' and 'The Gravy Train' classes of The KCD.

The difficulty that controllers have is that they cannot have true relationships with people. The only relationships that appear to work are those on the controller's terms. This means they are most likely to end up with a compliant person that 'cannot say NO,' to their 'cannot hear NO.'

3. The non-responsive: 'Can't say YES'

The non-responsive cannot say 'YES.' This means that they avoid responsibility in life. The underlying belief is that it is not their job. The non-responsive may have learnt this form of behavior from lax parenting, where the child was given no responsibility. The exact opposite childhood influences of not being able to say 'NO' can result in adult rebellion and a non-responsive.

Non-responsive individuals have extremely rigid boundaries and do not work well in teams or relationships. This form of boundary issue is common in 'The Gravy Train' class of The KCD.

4. The avoidant: 'Can't hear YES'

The avoidant sets boundaries against receiving care and help of others. The underlying belief structure of an avoidant is likely to be either 'I am not good enough' or 'There is only me.' This may have been created when there was a perceived insufficient emotional, physical, or financial help for a child.

To make matters worse, the avoidant tends to over help others, which accentuates their lack of support. The avoidant suffers from a lack of vulnerability in relationships and isolation. This form of boundary issue may be prevalent in 'The Jukebox' and 'The Dynamite' classes of The KCD.

Changing your boundaries; changing you

Different situations and individuals may well require a variety of boundary settings. As all human beings have their own distinct barriers, then relating to each other can look more like a dance. If two individuals have very tight fortifications then there will be little sharing. However, if one has tight boundaries and the other person's are lax, then this can result in the former taking advantage of the latter. Therefore, flexibility is crucial in managing the outer limits of healthy relationships. In general, it is best to start with a boundary setting somewhere in the middle. The diagram below shows the four extremities of this.

Can't say NO					Can't hear NO
Can't say YES					Can't hear YES

The management of boundary issues:

Observation is the first step in managing any area of an individual's behavior. Then there is practice, more observation, and tinkering, followed by more practice.

Change of boundaries will affect the individual's psyche, as it will often be different than an underlying belief structure. Also the people interacting with this individual will have to work out the new dynamic. They may embrace or fight this.

Learning to set new boundaries is like learning to ride a bicycle. It takes time, feels strange, has its moments of pain, but ultimately becomes natural and easy. Below is a suggested list of how to change boundary settings.

1. Observe boundaries in different relationships.
2. Practice altering boundaries in different settings.
3. Observe the feelings and results of altering boundaries.
4. Challenge those feelings if they are not helping in changing boundary settings. CBT can be useful for this.
5. Treat the underlying inner monologue that fuels the initial boundary settings. This can be done with inner child psychoanalysis or PSYCHOLOGICALSURGERY.

6. Treat the underlying KCD class as discussed elsewhere in this book.

7. Then go back to step 1.

Examples of boundary changes and their results

1. The compliant: 'Can't say NO'

A compliant that previously could not say 'NO' may feel guilty when they do this. Others may fight against their choice of 'NO' because they are so used to all their demands being met. If the compliant maintains healthy boundaries, they will either lose unhealthy relationships or have them redefined. The individual may start saying 'NO' to everything. This is likely to be a short-lived phase and is normal in the learning process.

2. The controller: 'Can't hear NO'

The controller may at first feel cheated that they are accepting 'NO' from others. Those they interact with may consider that the behavior change is just part of a larger manipulation. They tend to get little credit for this 'monumental' change because others view their new behavior as normal. To maintain healthy boundaries, a controller needs to address the underlying belief structure that they are worthless or unlovable.

3. The non-responsive: 'Can't say YES'

The non-responsive may well feel put upon by saying 'YES.' Others may start to take advantage, or feel that the non-responsive's 'YES' has strings attached. The non-responsive may also feel vulnerable saying 'YES,' even in protected environments, and the key is to feel love for others and safety for themselves.

4. The avoidant: 'Can't hear YES'

The avoidant, who allows love and help into their life, may well release a lot of stored up emotion. Allowing the 'YES' may break the curse that they are either unlovable or unworthy. Tears and anger may ensue initially, which the avoidant and others may be frightened of. Also the avoidant may become disappointed when they accept help and do not get it. The key is to work through this with others (including professionals) to slowly open up, deal with the stored emotions, and accept that they are as worthy and lovable as everyone else.

Table of likely boundary issues and suggestions for overcoming them, within The KCD:

Class of depression	Possible boundary issue	Explanation	Suggested ways of improving
The Mountain Mule	compliant	There is an inner belief, that you are responsible for others. Hence you cannot say NO.	Start saying NO to anything you feel resentful about. You may at first feel guilty but continue making choices. Is it really true, that you have to help anyone that asks?
The Jukebox	controller / non-responsive	Your addiction to your thoughts often translates into you expecting others to do as you wish. You cannot hear a NO. You may well have some aspects of the opposite cannot say YES.	The Jukebox controller / non-responsive Your addiction to your thoughts often translates into you expecting others to do as you wish. You cannot hear a NO. You may well have some aspects of the opposite cannot say YES. The key here is to get present to your thoughts and the fact that they are just one opinion of many. Work on a compromise of helping others and being helped. You may find at first that people doubt your sincerity in this change and that you feel used when.
The Stuck Trapeze	non-responsive / avoidant	You are stuck because you cannot hear a YES from the world and others. You also cannot say YES to the world otherwise. Feeling trapped you are fearful of what YES might bring.	It is time to focus on what you do want and take the leap of life. Be in love with life, allow help of others as well as be a yes to yourself. Stop procrastinating and just say YES.
A Loss Reaction -if excessive	avoidant / controller	An excessive loss reaction may occur when you cannot hear NO from the universe and others and accept the loss. You may also have excessive grief reaction if you are unwilling to accept practical and emotional help from others. Therefore you cannot hear.	Work through the grief reaction as explained in earlier chapters. At some point you need to accept what has happened, why not now? Allow others to help you. You are worth it.
The Dynamite	avoidant	Your emotions have not been released over the years because you do not accept help from others. You cannot hear a YES.	You need help to release your emotions as discussed in previous chapters. Start saying YES to when people offer to help, this is a strength.
Naturally Deficient	nil specific	nil specific	nil specific
The Gravy Train	controller / non-responsive	You are controlling the situation by remaining depressed. In fact depression may be the way to avoid hearing a NO. It is also a way to avoid saying YES to life and responsibility.	It is time to see the control you truly have in your world. You have more personal power than you wish to believe. If acknowledged, then you can start to train yourself to say YES to life and to hear NO from others.
The Princess and the Pauper	combination of controller and compliant	You fluctuate from one belief structure to another. On one end of the spectrum you feel unworthy and cannot say NO. On the other extreme you find it difficult to hear a NO from others.	Each extreme boundary position needs to be isolated and worked on seperately. One needs to hear NO and to say YES, the other needs to say NO and hear a YES.
The Empty and Overflowing Tank	nil specific	nil specific	nil specific
Medical	nil specific	nil specific	nil specific

139

An example of boundary setting:

Claire, 30, had worked for the Metropolitan Police Service for 10 years. Initially she had enjoyed her job, but for the past year she had become anxious and depressed. After a minor complaint had been made about her attitude, she had broken down and cried. It transpired that she could not say 'NO' to any request and was hence exhausted.

At first she began to observe where she said 'YES,' but felt resentful. She would say 'YES' to all the extra shifts she was asked to do by her colleagues. There was a 'YES' to staying in the police force, when she wanted to become a gardener. She even muttered 'YES' every time her ungrateful younger sister wanted a lift.

Claire was shocked by her reticence to say 'NO' and decided that it was time to change. She first refused to do extra shift work. Then she said 'NO' to giving her 17 year old sister a lift to a party. Her sister screamed at her for being 'selfish.' For Claire had had driving lessons from her father, but her sister could not, because he was dead. Claire felt guilty for saying 'NO' but continued in her boundary alterations.

Claire was surprised by her huge sense of guilt and underwent Inner Child Psychoanalysis. She discovered an underlying belief that she 'was not important.' As Claire was growing up, her mother suffered from severe alcoholism. As she could not cope very well, Claire was expected to do many of the household chores and to look after her sister. This had got worse after her father's death about 10 years previously.

Claire was diagnosed with 'The Mountain Mule' class of The KCD. She began to write copious 'should lists' and underwent CBT to challenge her thoughts – one of which was that it was up to her to look after her mother, irrespective of the latter's behavior.

Claire told her mother it was time that she looked after herself. Her mother threatened that if Claire did not help her in the house, then she might die because she would not eat. Claire refused to visit. For the next 3 months she continued to say 'NO' to her mother and sister.

Claire decided that she was being a little harsh on her family and began saying 'YES' again. This time it was her choice. Her mother and sister began to thank her for the subsequent help she gave. She also enrolled in horticultural night classes.

Chapter 19

Feeding Your Happiness

Having a healthy diet is extremely important for both general health and in the management of depression. General principles of an optimum diet include:

1.   Constant energy levels, therefore small regular meals.

2.   Eat sufficient fiber, so that you have regular bowel function. This can be found in fruit, vegetables, and cereals such as oatmeal.

3.   Ensure enough good fats such as fish oils in your diet. Reduce saturated fats.

4.   Make sure there are ample vitamins and minerals – this is best achieved by eating at least five portions of different colored fruits and vegetables a day. There is debate in the medical world as to whether taking vitamin supplements is beneficial. In my experience, taking one good multivitamin a day is likely to be helpful.

5.   Avoid foods that may induce intolerances – many processed foods are particularly prone to do this.

6.   Foods that cause cravings are probably bad for you.

7.   Avoid foods that may contain hormones or antibiotics – these can be especially prevalent in non-organic meats.

8.   Have long-acting carbohydrates that break down slowly, rather than simple sugars that cause peaks and troughs in your blood glucose and energy levels.

9.   Reduce or avoid stimulants such as coffee, as these produce peaks and troughs of energy and can affect the adrenal glands.

10.   Minimize alcohol intake, avoiding binge drinking in particular.

11. Ensure good hydration. This can be achieved with high quantities of certain fruits or drinking plenty of water each day.

Below are some deeper explanations of why the food that you ingest can affect your mood, and advice on how that can be changed.

1. Let your energy levels be like a flat meadow and not the Swiss Alps

Eating sugary foods causes a sudden spike in blood glucose levels. This then causes a hormone called insulin to be released in the body. This in turn facilitates the sugar in the blood to go into the cells, and to be either stored or turned into fat. This results in a low blood sugar level and therefore a craving for something sweet. The individual then eats a quick acting sugary substance and the cycle repeats itself. The level of sugar in a person's body goes up and down, like a mountain range. This has a number of problems.

1.   Increases insulin release – which increases fat and the possibility of diabetes.

2.   The changes in sugar levels cause stress in the body and release of stress-inducing hormones.

3.   Lack of a constant level of sugar reduces general energy, concentration, and mood.

Having a stable sugar level is important in maintaining a happy mind. I suggest eating long-acting carbohydrates, such as brown rice or pasta, and wholemeal bread, in preference to sugar in drinks, chocolate bars, and processed food that has high amounts of sugar. Replace these cravings with fruit instead. Many very healthy people significantly reduce all processed carbohydrates. They may have diets that contain fruits, vegetables, nuts, pulses, fish, and lean meat.

2. You need to oil your brain.

Studies have shown links between low cholesterol and depression. This does not mean, I believe, we should be increasing our cholesterol levels. However, it is important to have a good level of fat in our diets. More evidence is emerging that suggests it is the ratio of the types of fat that you eat that is also important. Many diets are high in omega 9 and 6 fats, found in meats and processed foods. However, levels of omega-3 (found in fish oils and various cereal crops) can be paradoxically low. I believe many diets need to increase omega-3. The easiest way to achieve this is to take fish oil supplements or increase intake of fish.

3. Get more than your five a day

Despite the fact that many of us are eating more food than ever, we may not be acquiring enough essential vitamins and minerals. There are many foods that are high in calorie counts but low in goodness. Processed foods and fast foods are particularly liable in this regard. Therefore, eating AT LEAST FIVE portions of different colored fruit and vegetables a day is very important. I would also recommend a good quality multivitamin as well.

4. Treat yourself to an expert

What we eat and drink enters our body and forms all our cells. Therefore, we are a product of the food we eat. Individuals require different diets depending on genetic factors, food intolerances, blood grouping, age, and health. I recommend the help of a good nutritionist for all individuals with depression, if they can practically do this. This help may be as important as seeing a therapist. The reason for this is different foods can have profound effects on various people. They can:

1. Change the hormone balance of a person, which can increase depression. Examples include, depression caused by male low testosterone, which can be worsened by the estrogen affect in high quantities of soya products. Some diets increase release of stress hormones, whereas other products may inhibit hormones such as thyroxin.

2. Lack of essential vitamins and minerals can directly reduce an individual's mood.

3. Food that causes intolerance reduces the energy of an individual and hence can cause depression.

4. Being overweight can cause pain, and the fat cells may hold onto emotion.

5. Being unhappy with the shape of the body can often translate into a negative mood.

If weight management is an important part of a new healthy lifestyle, then joining a club such as Weight Watchers can be extremely helpful. Many programs give both moral support and calorie reducing tools. However, they do not give specific dietary advice for an individual. They certainly do not target specific advice for those suffering depression.

Many individuals feel that they need support because they have an obsessive eating or drinking problem. For them a peer-led 12-step program can be useful. These are run by the participants themselves, and work in helping each other through practical and spiritual steps, in order to gain control over an addiction. There are many of these groups in big cities all around the globe. The local meetings are usually easily found on their websites. Examples include Overeaters Anonymous and

Alcoholics Anonymous. If you choose to attend these meetings, I suggest you mention this to your doctor or therapist first.

Chapter 20

Guide to Helpful Processes and Therapeutic Substances

Within this chapter is a list of various processes and therapeutic substances which are useful in the treatment of depression. Many of these have been discussed in earlier chapters. The explanations are brief and reflect my own understanding of the issues. I have limited the number of entries to those that are well-known, either generally or to myself. This approach is not intended to negate many other processes and therapeutic substances which may be extremely appropriate for a person's depression.

As discussed in the earlier chapters, each class of The KCD requires different approaches for treatment. An example would be that for 'The Mountain Mule' class of depression. A treatment that works on the conscious level, such as CBT, is often very helpful, whereas 'The Jukebox' may require a deeper approach, such as NLP. Even if one of the following options does not obviously fit an individual's class of The KCD, it may still be beneficial. You will need to discuss with your doctor or mental health professional the treatment options that you have chosen.

Simple Options

1. No obvious active measures

An individual may choose to make no obvious treatment plan for their depression, or may decide to instigate a plan of action at different time intervals or at various levels of severity. Others may wish to sit with a diagnosis for a while before they feel able to commit to treatment.

Individuals have the right to choose to take action or not. This is best respected as few treatments work if the person does not wish to partake in them.

In some cases, the mere act of recognizing that there is a problem can be of great benefit. In itself this knowledge may be sufficient to begin a non-specific healing process.

2. Time to rest and think – avoid the overflowing tank of life

Being idle can allow the mind and body to relax. Many modern lifestyles are so hectic that an individual never has time to recuperate. Being idle is often avoided by people because there can be an underlying social convention that they are either boring or lazy. However, many successful people create hours of idleness in their diaries in order for their minds to function at a high level. Time spent doing nothing can be extremely beneficial. It may facilitate a clearer mind, where answers to personal questions may emerge, and emotions can calm down.

3. Sleep

The subconscious has a much higher ability to process information than the conscious mind. Therefore, issues and emotions that would 'swamp' the conscious mind are best left to the deeper processing powers of the subconscious. The conscious mind needs to be switched off for the subconscious to work fully; this is achieved during sleep. Lack of sleep will inhibit the mind's ability to process information. This leaves unresolved thoughts and emotions in the conscious mind, which causes confusion.

Sleep can be as curative as many of the other treatment options that are discussed in this chapter. For a number of my patients, I suggest that they take a whole day or weekend off to sleep. In many cases, they feel that they do not have the time because of work or family commitments. However, if the importance of sleep is fully recognized then arrangements can be put into place.

Oversleeping may be a symptom of some individuals' depression. Often the sleep is poor and the time spent in bed is used to ruminate on negative aspects of their life. This is particularly so of 'The Jukebox' class of The KCD. Those individuals suffering from a severe form of 'The Stuck Trapeze' may also spend huge amounts of time in bed, in order to avoid moving forward with their life. For these individuals, a bed restriction is important. Although each person can choose a certain bedtime allowance, I normally suggest that 9 hours is sufficient. (Some scientific research suggests that a full cycle of sleep takes 3 hours. For the healthiest patterns, we need to sleep for multiples of this.)

Particular issues that can help in healthy sleep are:

Exercise earlier in the day.

Avoid stimulants and caffeinated drinks after lunchtime.

Eat a small but satisfying dinner.

Limit sugars in the evening.

Reduce stimulation such as television or computer use an hour before bedtime.

Have a dark, tidy bedroom.

Relax by either reading or listening to music.

Write a diary for the day.

Drink calming teas such as chamomile.

If a sleeping pattern is extremely difficult to regulate, then sleeping

149

tablets or herbal remedies can be used. Many preparations are addictive, so use should be limited as much as possible. In general a 3-day course of sleeping tablets is sufficient.

4. Getting away

Getting away from your current environment can facilitate a healing period of reflection. For when a person can look at their lives from afar, emotions and stresses reduce.

A break may include a visit to the countryside, a pampering holiday, or just time in the sun and being surrounded by nature. Traveling alone may have its benefits, as it can allow issues to clarify. However, it may also lead to mental rumination and loneliness. In contrast, visiting loved ones can facilitate a greater feeling of connection and worth.

Individuals who wish for company on their break, but have no obvious partner to accompany them, may find a group activity holiday to be an excellent option. There are many of these available and include a diverse array of activities, from yoga and painting to sports and walking.

A break away can also facilitate an increase in sunshine and exercise, which are extremely important for overcoming depression.

5. Pampering

For those individuals that suffer from a lack of self worth then self-pampering can be extremely therapeutic. This is particularly important for 'The Mountain Mule' category of The KCD. There are many ways to achieve this, and some examples include buying and wearing nice clothes and having a haircut or manicure. When the outside of a person looks good, then this has a positive effect on the inside.

Pampering can also include massages, listening to great music, going to the theatre or cinema, and eating at a wonderful restaurant.

Medications

Symptoms of depression **may** respond well to either short- or long-term medications. This is so for all types of The KCD but is often vital in the 'Naturally Deficient' class. 'The Prince/ss and the Pauper' also has a high likelihood that medication will be used in its treatment.

Decisions regarding use of medication need to be made between a patient and their doctor on an individual basis. I do believe, however, that in Western medicine depression medication is overused. This is a major problem because:

1. The responsibility for healing depression goes from patient to doctor and drug.

2. There are increased side effects of medication.

3. There can be a mind numbing effect of the medication.

4. The medication does not result in a long-term cure for many individuals.

5. Depression can act as a warning system that change needs to occur in a person's life. Using medication may divert the individual from this purpose.

Despite my belief in limiting medication, I have given a snapshot of the common classes of them below. I have used my own experience and accessible data to compile the following details. The information is far from complete, and it is vital that if considering their use you discuss this with your doctor first. A more comprehensive understanding of these substances, including side effects and conditions where they are contra indicated, can be found in the pharmaceutical companies' information sheets and websites, and data compiled in sources such as the British National Formulary (BNF).

1. Sleeping tablets and tablets to sedate and reduce anxiety (anxiolytics)

Sleeping tablets can help in regulating sleeping patterns. They tend to help a patient fall asleep but often do not keep a person asleep. These medications include drugs such as zopiclone and nitrazepam. They are best used on a short-term basis because long-term use may lead to addiction. I tend to suggest three nights of use initially, in order to regulate sleep patterns. Side effects may include sleepiness, fatigue, motor impairment, and headaches.

For individuals where staying asleep may be an issue, the use of longer acting medication, such as low dose amitriptyline, may be more beneficial in gaining a full night's sleep. Side effects can include headaches, dry mouth, erectile dysfunction, and weight changes.

Drugs used to reduce anxiety symptoms include medications such as diazepam (Valium), lorazepam, and propranolol.

Diazepam and lorazepam are addictive in their nature and should be used with great caution. Both reduce anxiety symptoms and muscle tension. Short-term use can be extremely helpful, especially for treatment of panic attacks.

Another option to reduce symptoms of anxiety, such as palpitations, is a group of drugs called beta-blockers. An example of these is a drug called propranolol. These beta-blockers reduce heart rate and can therefore calm a patient. Side effects include wheezing, lightheadedness, and fluid retention. It should be avoided in asthma sufferers and in cases of heart failure. Propranolol can be used short- or long-term, as it does not have the addictive nature of the other tablets in this section.

2. Antidepressants

A – The SSRIs (selective serotonin reuptake inhibitors)

SSRIs include drugs such as Prozac (fluoxetine), citalopram, and Seroxat. They are the commonest medications currently prescribed for depression. They work by reducing the breakdown of a chemical in the brain called serotonin, and hence increasing its level at the nerve endings. This is believed to increase mood.

They may have an immediate effect, but often it takes 3 weeks to really start to work and 3 months to reach maximal effect. My exception to this rule is in the 'Naturally Deficient' class of The KCD; a positive effect may occur in days, rather than weeks.

Side effects include changes in sleep patterns, stomach upsets, and altered bowel function. Many of these happen in the first 3 weeks and then resolve. Paradoxically, many doctors feel that the worse the side effects initially, the better the result of medication. If you do get side effects, though, you need to discuss this with your doctor as soon as possible. Liver function problems and stomach ulcers can occur with these medications, and may preclude individuals from using them.

Many clinicians keep an individual on this medication for 4–6 months after the symptoms of depression are alleviated. It is believed that when the brain is accustomed to a certain level of serotonin, it will maintain it. It does this by increasing its own production after the medication is ceased. It is standard procedure to reduce medication slowly, over weeks and months, in order to give the brain time to acclimatize.

In the 'Naturally Deficient,' it is usual that longer-term medication is required.

B – SSRIs and noradrenaline receptor

Though serotonin appears to be the main brain chemical to affect mood, low levels of another neurotransmitter called noradrenaline can also have a negative effect on mood.

Medications such as Effexor (venlafaxine) are thought to increase levels of both neurotransmitters. They are stronger than the SSRIs alone. They tend to be prescribed in either severe or resistant cases of depression. Side effects include constipation, nausea, and weakness.

Tricyclic antidepressants

Before the SSRIs were available, the 'tricyclics' were the mainstay of medication treatment in depression. They have a much higher sedative effect than the SSRIs and are of particular use if lack of sleep is a problem.

Doctors also view them as being safer in relation to heart problems, and they are therefore used more in elderly patients. However, the increase in drowsiness is believed to increase risk of falling.

Side effects include dry mouth, blurred vision, drowsiness, and tremors. Typical medications are called dothiepin and amitriptyline.

C – Monoamine oxidase inhibitors (MAOIs), including St. John's Wort

These medications are infrequently used as they interact with many other medications, including the contraceptive pill, and foods such as cheeses and grapefruits. Foods containing tyramine and tryptophan need to be avoided because they can set up severe interactions with these drugs.

As MAOIs can have severe side-effects, they are often used as a last resort measure. There are newer medications in this class that are available in skin patch form. This reduces problems in the gut.

The active ingredient in the herb St. John's Wort is a MAOI. Therefore, similar precautions need to be taken as above, if using this over the counter remedy. This is despite the fact that St. John's Wort uses a lower dose of MAOI than many of the pharmaceutical preparations. Some studies have shown that St. John's Wort is as effective as some of the SSRIs in treatment of mild depression.

D – Lithium

This medication has been shown to help depressive symptoms, especially in the diagnosis of bipolar disorders. It can be extremely useful in these cases, but has a number of side effects. These include shakiness, thirst, diarrhea, drowsiness, and weakness. The drug may also become dangerously toxic in the body, causing symptoms of ringing in the ears, shakiness, blurred vision, and seizures. If any of these symptoms occur, then a doctor needs to be informed straight away.

3. Other medication

If depression shows psychotic symptoms (such as hallucinations or delusional thinking), or does not respond to the above medications, psychiatrists may add in anti-psychotic medications. Examples of these are risperidone and olanzapine.

Supplements from health food shops

(*http://www.health.com/health/article/0,,20411993_1,00.html*)

There are many supplements available in health food shops to help a person's mood. In general there is mixed evidence supporting their effectiveness. They may also have side effects, so that it is important to discuss use of these preparations with your doctor. A few of the common supplements are listed below.

1 – 5-Hydroxytryptophan (5HT)

5-Hydroxytryptophan, also known as 5HT, is sold as a supplement in health food shops. It is an amino acid that occurs naturally in foods and is converted to serotonin. Therefore, it is believed to increase the brain's serotonin level, and hence alleviate symptoms of depression. Due to a lack of scientific research there are limited details of potential side effects and effectiveness.

2 – S-adenosylmethionine (SAM-e)

S-adenosylmethionine (SAM-e) is a naturally occurring compound that increases serotonin levels. There is some evidence that it improves depression symptoms, especially when injected. There are a number of side effects associated with SAM-e; in particular it can exacerbate mania or hypomania in people with bipolar disorder.

3 – Omega-3s

Omega-3s contain polyunsaturated fatty acids EPA and DHA, which are the main ingredients in fish oil. Some research on omega-3s and mood disorders is encouraging, but it remains unclear just how effective they are. They have few side effects and have cardiovascular and other health benefits.

Psychological options – conscious treatments

1. Counseling

Counseling works on the conscious level. This process facilitates an individual to unburden their thoughts and emotions. The counselor may give feedback on these or avoid interrupting an individual's conversation. In this way, a counselor acts as a non-judgmental and safe sounding-board.

Releasing what is most on an individual's mind can be extremely cathartic. Sometimes the therapy session is the only place that a person feels safe to fully express him or herself.

This form of therapy can be particularly useful for those that tend to keep their thoughts and emotions bottled inside. For it permits free expression. 'The Dynamite' and 'The Mountain Mule' classes of The KCD can particularly benefit from this.

Counseling can have a negative effect in the treatment of 'The Jukebox' and 'The Gravy Train' classes of The KCD, for conversations can be rooted in past thoughts and events. There is also the risk of going over the same thing again and again, which can be part of an addiction. This reinforces their negative habitual behavior pattern.

2. Life coaching

Strictly speaking this is not a form of therapy, but can be extremely useful. It works fully on the conscious level by sorting out all the practical aspects of an individual's life.

It is very useful for those that have specific, tangible challenges; overcoming them can reduce stresses and concerns. It can also be very effective in helping an individual to create the future that they truly desire, by ensuring the actions required are put into place.

In many ways life coaching can help everybody. It keeps a person on track with the practical aspect of their life. This often leads to a greater feeling of control and a better mood.

A life coach can be particularly useful for 'The Mountain Mule,' 'Loss Reaction,' and 'The Stuck Trapeze' classes of The KCD.

3. Psychoanalysis

Psychoanalysis is the process in which an individual's subconscious is analyzed. Popularized initially by the paradigm shifting geniuses, such as Sigmund Freud and Carl Jung, it has many current forms.

All variations take into account the principle that the human subconscious is programmed from a young age. These 'programs' then form personalities, habits, and underlying belief structures. By understanding these programs, an individual can then make sense of why they have certain current feelings and emotions. Interventions can then be undertaken to change those on-going patterns.

In the building of an individual's psyche, many influences occur. By the time a person reaches adulthood, there are the understandings of the world as an adult, a child, and as a society or family unit. Each understanding brings a different voice to that person. In general there are at least three competing 'voices' in a human adult's head. These are the adult, the child, and society.

Many belief structures are formalized in childhood, and therefore much psychoanalysis is required at this stage. The childhood voice is often frightened and emotionally needy, and requires 'parenting' from the adult individual. This form of therapy is often called **Inner Child Psychoanalysis.**

Other therapies look at dealing with the voice of society around the individual. The greatest influence in this area is often that of the parents. When this 'voice' is particularly strong, then a person does not lead his or her own life. Instead, they follow the instructions of their parents as if they were still guiding their life. This can occur even in 80 and 90 year olds.

The main aim of psychotherapy is for an individual to understand why they have a particular belief structure. This can then be challenged if it is not in keeping with that of a happy and healthy adult.

These techniques work on the subconscious. They are particularly useful for 'The Jukebox,' 'The Stuck Trapeze,' 'The Dynamite,' 'The Prince/ss and the Pauper,' and if excessive or on-going, the 'Loss Reaction' classes of The KCD. For 'The Mountain Mule' psychotherapy can uncover the underlying belief of why they cannot say 'NO.'

4. Cognitive Behavioral Therapy (CBT)

Cognitive Behavioral Therapy works on the conscious level. It encourages the individual to look at the relationship between their thoughts, emotions, and action in creating the results in their lives. It then facilitates in the breaking of old patterns of behavior and creating new empowering ones.

In a nutshell, CBT works on the following understanding:

Thoughts become **feelings** that produce **actions** that produce **results**, which in turn produce reinforced thoughts and feelings.

Thoughts

↓

Feelings

↓

Actions

↓

Results

↓

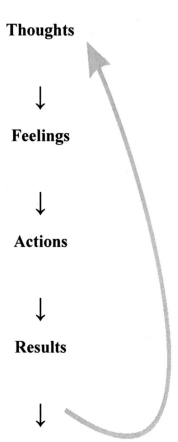

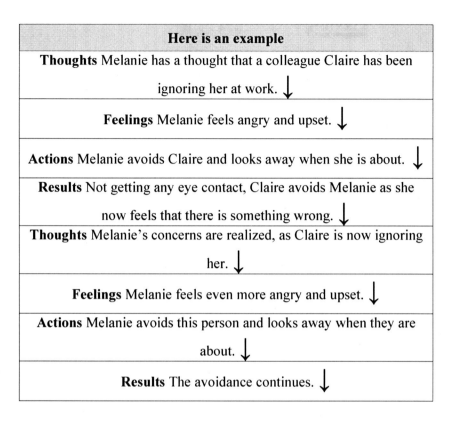

Here is an example
Thoughts Melanie has a thought that a colleague Claire has been ignoring her at work. ↓
Feelings Melanie feels angry and upset. ↓
Actions Melanie avoids Claire and looks away when she is about. ↓
Results Not getting any eye contact, Claire avoids Melanie as she now feels that there is something wrong. ↓
Thoughts Melanie's concerns are realized, as Claire is now ignoring her. ↓
Feelings Melanie feels even more angry and upset. ↓
Actions Melanie avoids this person and looks away when they are about. ↓
Results The avoidance continues. ↓

It was suggested to Melanie that despite her thoughts and feelings to the contrary, she could change her actions. She was encouraged to smile at Claire and ask her if there was anything wrong. Melanie did this. To her surprise, Melanie replied that she thought Claire did not like her because of her lack of eye contact. The end result was a better work environment. In other words, to get a different result, we have to put in a different action.

CBT works at any level of thoughts, feelings, or action. This process may be particularly useful for 'The Mountain Mule,' 'Loss Reaction,' and 'The Stuck Trapeze' forms of The KCD. It does not tackle the deeper issues of 'The Jukebox' class of The KCD.

5. Primal Therapy*

Primal Therapy can be helpful in releasing both the physical and emotional pains that are stored in the body. The Primal therapist is to help the patient to re-experience and express the pain that was repressed, with full connection to the source of the traumatic event, or painful prolonged situation, that caused the repression in the first place**. This therapy is particularly useful for 'The Dynamite' class of The KCD.

For more information: *'Primal Therapy: What It Is and What It Is Not,' by Réal Beaulieu, MA, MFT, Primal Therapist (written in 1986, revised in 1988 with important footnote: year 2000) http://primal-page.com/beau.htm.

**There have been mixed reviews regarding primal therapy. As the process can release an enormous amount of emotion, a number of experts have suggested that only highly experienced therapists perform this technique.

Psychological options – subconscious treatments

All these processes can be particularly useful for 'The Dynamite,' 'The Jukebox,' 'Loss Reaction,' 'The Mountain Mule,' 'The Prince/ss and the Pauper,' 'The Gravy Train,' and 'The Stuck Trapeze' classes of The KCD.

1. Hypnosis

Hypnosis works by relaxing the patient to such a degree that the conscious mind switches off. In this state, the subconscious mind is open to either give information or to be reprogrammed directly. Past, present and future programs can be created. Hypnosis is particularly useful in reducing compulsive behavior, such as smoking or overeating.

2. Neuro Linguistic Programming (NLP)

NLP works by using words and images to create a new subconscious program. It allows new empowering beliefs about life. In many cases, a few sessions suffice to create this new program. The premise of NLP is that the subconscious stores information from the five senses. However, the subconscious does not recognize the difference between 'true' senses and imagined ones. By flooding the subconscious using the five senses, a new program can be created.

3. Emotional Freedom Technique (EFT)

This technique combines the fact that certain points on our body surface are connected to our brain's subconscious. Therefore, by tapping on them, new programs can be instilled in a similar way that Pavlov trained his dogs. It can be particularly useful for stress release, as well as changing deep emotional patterns.

4. Eye Movement Desensitization and Reprocessing (EMDR)

EMDR involves recalling a stressful past event and 'reprogramming' the memory in the light of a positive, self-chosen belief, while using rapid eye movements. In a typical EMDR therapy session the patient focuses on traumatic memories, and tracks the therapist's moving finger with their eyes, as it moves back and forth across their visual fields. Though not fully understood why, this process helps to dissociate the picture of the event and the emotions that are attached to it. When this occurs, the event can be examined from a more detached perspective, somewhat like watching a movie of what happened.

One reason this dissociation may occur is because our eyes move in different directions during storing, remembering and creating information. Imagine the storing of an event is like crocheting a piece of material. The whole event is the combination of all the strands of different colored wools that you use. Our eye movements may act as the needles that pull the strands together. These strands are the visions, sounds, feelings, and emotions. Repeating the image of the event again and having the eyes move is akin to the needles unpicking the individual pieces of wool. Therefore, the piece of 'wool' that represents emotion is separated from the vision. Then the vision can be worked on and altered without any interference from the enormous emotional input.

This form of therapy can be particularly useful for 'The Jukebox' sub-class of The KCD called post-traumatic stress disorder (PTSD).

5. PsychologicalSurgery (PS)

PsychologicalSurgery (PS) is the new highly precise technique for focusing the energy of an individual in the direction of an empowering future. It combines a number of other psychological approaches to program the subconscious with the desired goals, then regresses to childhood to remove the specific lifelong blocks that would hold that dream back. It uses a combination of NLP, Inner Child Psychoanalysis, the emotional regression of 'The Journey Process,' and aspects of CBT.

The procedure usually occurs in one session, which can last many hours. The personalized subconscious program is then reinforced with a daily taped meditation. PS was created by myself over the last 10 years and has been successfully used in the worlds of sport and business, and for the treatment of depression.

See www.drnickkrasner.com

Other treatments

1. Light Box Therapy

Used in the therapy of Seasonal Affective Disorder (SAD), Light Box Therapy uses a very bright fluorescent light of at least 10,000 lux, in order to mimic sunlight. In the early morning, an individual sits 2–3 feet away from the light box, without looking at it. They do this for approximately 30 minutes in order to simulate daybreak. The treatment can cause eyestrain, headaches, and occasionally mania. Any individual who has sensitivity to light should avoid this therapy.

For more information:

http://www.ncbi.nlm.nih.gov/pubmedhealth/PMH0002499/

2. Group work

This can use many techniques of counseling or CBT, but is done in a group. It has the advantage of encouraging feelings of belonging. It also highlights that what one person is going through is shared by many.

'Self help' psychological options

1. 'The Journey Process'

'The Journey Process' was developed by Brandon Bays to facilitate emotional and physical self-healing. Using a relaxation technique it works back through the emotions to discover and 'heal' those first moments the emotions were created.

It is particularly useful in 'The Dynamite,' 'The Jukebox,' and 'Loss Reaction' classes of The KCD.

For more information go to *http://www.thejourney.com*

2. The Work

'The Work' was created by Byron Katie to identify and question the thoughts that cause fear and depression. It works on the conscious level

165

in a similar way to CBT. The work asks four questions in regard to any of our thoughts. They are:

1. Is it true?

2. Can I absolutely know it's true?

3. How do I react when I believe this thought?

4. Who would I be without the thought?

By working through these questions, it is believed that a clearing occurs in the mind. Sometimes an individual has to cycle through the four questions many times in order to clear mental brain patterns. These processes can be particularly useful for the 'The Dynamite,' 'The Mountain Mule,' 'The Prince/ss and the Pauper,' and 'The Stuck Trapeze' classes of The KCD.

More information is at the website www.thework.com

3. The 'should' list and 'shoulding' yourself

'Shoulding' yourself was first termed by the psychologist Clayton Barbeau, and is the automatic thought that you or someone else is obliged to do something. This is an unreasoned response and often leads to guilt. There are three classes of 'SHOULD,' which are:

'I should' – personal 'obligations.'

'You should' – what you feel other people's obligations are.

'It should' – how you think an organization, country, society, or the world should act.

Psychologists have worked with 'I should' in various ways. One is simply to write down all the 'I shoulds' in order to uncover them. This is a 'should list.' Then you can deal with these beliefs by rationally deciding if they actually are true. The four questions in Byron Katie's 'The Work' are particularly good for this.

Many psychologists believe that when an individual thinks 'I should,' they would benefit from challenging it. Simply changing the term to 'I choose' gives a person more mental freedom and personal power; for when a person 'chooses' it gives them the option to say 'NO.'

'Should lists' are particularly useful for 'The Mountain Mule' class of The KCD.

PART 4

PUTTING THE KCD INTO ACTION

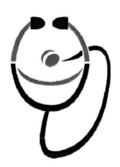

Chapter 21

Putting It Into Practice

It is now time to put all the previous information into an action plan. A daily ritual can then be created, which will help to consistently pull you from a negative to a positive mindset.

In formulating this plan we will combine all aspects covered earlier in the book. These topics include:

How to diagnose your class of depression of The KCD

The treatment options for each class of The KCD

Explanation of what these treatments are

How to grade the severity of depression on a day-to-day basis

Essential choices for a stable mood such as diet, exercise, sunlight, nature, love, purpose, and socializing

Learning to take responsibility without blame

Creating healthy boundaries

Tricks for getting out of a depressive mood

Remember: It is highly recommended to gain the help of a professional and a trusted friend or family member during this process.

Creating a plan of action

The plans most likely to work will simultaneously combine:

The healing of your past

The ability to become 'present'

The image of a positive future

The reason why it is important to combine the above processes is because the brain abhors a vacuum. If you work hard to remove negative mind patterns, then the brain will fill this void with 'something.' That 'something' will be the strongest available thought process. If you create a powerful future, then this may well become the mind pattern that is adopted on the subconscious. If this is not available, then the brain tends to recreate the negative mind pattern that you have just got rid of.

So practically, the following actions are required in creating the best plans:

A. Specific measures from The KCD.

B. Non-specific practices that create a happy mood.

C. Consciousness (being present to the NOW).

D. Creating your future.

Remember, the more you get used to feeling good, the more you will want to put positive actions into place. So start making a change today, even if your emotions are contrary to this. At some point, with continual action, your emotions will support your new way of being.

Practical aspects of an action plan

Below are four areas required to create a full action plan. I recommend that you write down or circle those actions that apply to you.

A. Specific Measures from The KCD

Below is a summary of the individual treatments suggested for the 10 classes of The KCD. You may wish to remind yourself of which class your depression belongs to. At the end of this section, I suggest writing down the appropriate treatment options that suit you best.

My form of depression is predominantly

....

I also have symptoms of the following class of depression

....

....

1. Suggested strategies to help 'THE MOUNTAIN MULE' class of The KCD:

1. Take stock of all you are doing.
2. Congratulate yourself on doing so much. YOU are a SUPERMAN or SUPERWOMAN.
3. Write a 'should' list.
   a. List 100+ things you are saying you should do.
   b. List of 'YOU SHOULD' for things you feel others 'should do'.
   c. List of 'IT SHOULD' for how you feel the world 'should be'.
4. Challenge these 'SHOULDs' using techniques such as:
   a. CBT.
   b. Life coaching.
   c. 'The Three Whats'.
   d. Byron Katie's 'The Work'.
5. For underlying beliefs from childhood, consider:
   a. Subconscious programming such as NLP or PS.
   b. Inner Child Psychoanalysis.
6. List your own minimum requirements in life, examples below, and prioritize them.
   a. Sleep.
   b. Diet.
   c. Time to self.

d. Fun.

e. Exercise.

7. Work out your boundaries with others.

    a. Read books on boundaries or go to seminars on boundary setting.

    b. Choose for yourself how much of yourself you wish to give to others.

    c. Practice saying 'No.' It will feel uncomfortable at first, but very empowering once you get accustomed to prioritizing your own needs.

8. Permit friends, families and colleagues to help you in your life.

2. Suggested strategies to help 'THE JUKEBOX' class of The KCD:

1. Understand that you are suffering from an addiction.

2. Therefore, understand in some ways you are powerless to overcome this alone.

3. You will need to forgive others (especially parents) and the younger you.

4. Start to train your mind to focus on positive thoughts, even when it does not want to or it feels strange to do so.

5. Observe your thoughts, such as 'Oh, I am complaining about the past again.'

6. Learn to say 'YES' to life and others.

7. GET HELP.

    a. Inner Child Psychoanalysis.

    b. Then get it reprogrammed on the subconscious via PS, NLP, or hypnosis.

8. Write a gratitude list every day (at least 10 things you are grateful for even if and when you do not feel like it).

9. Do regular positive mantras.

10. Imagine you have two CDs playing in 'The Jukebox' of your mind, one happy and one sad. The more you play a happy CD, the less the negative CD plays. Eventually the negative CD will disappear. Therefore keep focusing on positive thoughts.

11. Some people find that EFT or rapid eye movement therapies help with the addictive patterns.

12. At least three times every day bring yourself back into reality, by asking yourself: "What do I currently SEE, HEAR, FEEL, TASTE, and SMELL?"

3. Suggested strategies to help 'THE STUCK TRAPEZE' class of The KCD:

1. Write a list of pros and cons, for both staying where you are, and your new opportunities.

2. List the long term 'pain' you may have, if you do not jump from one trapeze to the next.

3. Look at any anxiety issues of 'change' from your past.

4. Get help with keeping yourself on task with creating the life you want.
   a. Life coach.
   b. Counselor.
   c. Friends/family.

5. Subconscious reprogramming may be helpful for underlying anxiety, via processes such as hypnosis, NLP, or PS.

6. If you cannot find the inciting moment for the anxiety, consider Inner Child Psychoanalysis.

7. Be prepared to make 'a leap of faith' in your life.

8. Learn techniques for becoming present as discussed earlier in the book.

4. Suggested strategies to help the 'LOSS REACTION' class of The KCD:

1. Understand that these symptoms are part of a natural process.

2. Allow yourself to work through each stage separately.

    a. Shock or disbelief – allow time to acclimatize to a new situation. Be gentle and kind to yourself.

    b. Denial – discuss with others what has happened, maybe a close friend, family, or a counselor.

    c. Bargaining – continue to get love and support from friends and family. If bargaining for long periods, you may need to learn to become present.

    d. Guilt – look at the situation from afar, to get a better understanding of what happened. 'The Three Whats' are particularly useful at this point:

        i.   WHAT is happening in reality?

        ii. So WHAT?

        iii. Now WHAT?

    e. Anger – allow the emotions out, either by talking or by screaming (in a safe place). Many people feel that punching a punch bag at the gym or pounding the streets for a run are extremely helpful.

f.   Depression – use of life coaches and Cognitive Behavioral Therapy are helpful in order to start to create a new future.

g.   Acceptance/hope – continue to work on your 'new' future as above.

3.   If symptoms are very severe, then CBT or occasionally medication may be indicated.

4.   The inability to move to the next stage of life can lead to 'The Stuck Trapeze' class of The KCD.

5. Suggested strategies to help 'THE DYNAMITE' class of The KCD:

1.   Acknowledge that you have emotional issues.

2.   Consider emotional workshops or treatments such as:

i.   'The Journey Process'.

ii.   Counseling.

iii.   Primal scream therapy.

iv.   PsychologicalSurgery.

3.   Find a safe place to dispel emotions such as anger, including:

i.   Boxing ring.

ii.   Yoga.

iii.   Gymnasium.

iv.   Climbing mountains.

4.   Treat physical pains.

5.   Lose weight if necessary.

6.   Write a letter to those with whom you are angry, expressing this emotion. DO NOT send it.

7.   Reduce substance use, with appropriate help from doctors or clinics.

6. Suggested strategies to help the 'NATURALLY DEFICIENT' class of The KCD:

1. Need to see doctor for treatment.
2. SSRIs likely the best drugs of choice.
3. Herbal medication may be useful such as 5HT, St. John's Wort, or SAM-E.
4. Understand that this form of depression is chemical and 'out of your control.'
5. Allow yourself to go on long-term replacement therapy.
6. Medication to be increased if necessary, until symptoms improve, as long as there are no side effects.
7. If necessary, titrate dose up or down to desired effect with help of your doctor.
8. If coming off long-term therapy, reduce slowly and if symptoms recur, go back on old dose of therapy.
9. Regular exercise.
10. A balanced healthy diet.
11. Sunlight.
12. Multivitamins are useful, especially including B complex.

7. Suggested strategies to help the 'THE GRAVY TRAIN' class of The KCD:

1. An expert is required in guiding the entire family.
2. Stop positive reinforcement of dramatic behavior.
3. Family therapy is useful, in order for the individual to be 'heard.'
4. Family therapy, as whole family is affected.

5. Boundary issues need to be worked on, so individual can hear 'NO' and say 'YES.'
6. Psychotherapy to reveal underlying fears.
7. Subconscious reprogramming of fears via hypnosis, NLP or PS.
8. Individual needs to learn to take personal responsibility.
9. Remove psychological or physical gain to being depressed.
10. A contract can be drawn up, in order to reinforce healthy behavior.

8. Suggested strategies to help 'THE PRINCE/SS AND THE PAUPER' class of The KCD:

1. Medication may be essential for this form of depression (as per your doctor).
2. Inner Child Psychoanalysis is advised to discover 'The Prince/ss' and 'The Pauper' separately.
3. PS, NLP, or hypnosis is useful for reprogramming each personality.
4. Each personality should be treated according to their class of The KCD.
5. Combination Therapy is required, in order to bring the 'Prince/ss' and the 'Pauper' together in a harmonious relationship.
6. Daily meditations, where both personalities interact with each other, are useful in maintaining a healthy relationship.
7. Different strategies created for manic and depressive phase of the condition:
   a. Have someone stop you spending large amounts when manic.

179

b. Do not make major decisions when manic.

c. Increase medication if necessary when manic.

d. Increase exercise when low.

e. Connect to others and do not isolate.

f. Eat regular, healthy meals.

g. If symptoms get worse, consult your doctor ASAP.

9a. Suggested strategies to help 'THE EMPTY TANK' class of The KCD:

1. Consider whether you are sufficient in the list below (for treatment see Chapter 10):

   a. Lack of sunlight.

   b. Lack of sleep.

   c. Taking depression-causing medication.

   d. Substance abuse, such as alcohol or marijuana.

   e. Poor nutrition.

   f. Lack of relaxation.

   g. Lack of love.

   h. Lack of touch.

   i. Lack of nature.

   j. Lack of passion.

   k. Lack of exercise.

   l. Lack of water.

2. See a doctor for blood tests and general check-up.

3. Receive professional nutritional advice.

4. Write a list of what makes you happy and commit to doing it.

5. A life coach or friend can be helpful in creating a weekly/daily routine that ensures good nutrition, sleep, exercise, and time for fun, passion, and love.

9b. Suggested strategies to help 'THE OVERFLOWING TANK' class of The KCD:

1. Forgive yourself for needing help.
2. Take a break.
3. Monitor your breathing – is it fast? Slow it down. The best way of doing this is to breathe in for 3 seconds, hold for 3 seconds and breathe out for 3 seconds.
4. Have relaxation time in your day; every day.
   a. Walking.
   b. Meditation.
   c. Yoga.
   d. Laughing with friends.
   e. Reading.
5. Have regular breaks away from work.
6. Allow yourself to be completely idle.
7. Have a priority list and deal with the issues that you are most concerned about.
8. Medication such as benzodiazepines and beta-blockers can be useful but can lead to addictions and have side effects.
9. Cut out all stimulants such as coffee, fizzy drinks, and sugary food.
10. Exercise can help burn up that stress like feeling.

11. If on going symptoms, you may need a life coach, counselor, or CBT to work on why you are getting so stressed and how to budget your time as listed above.

10. Suggested strategies to help the 'MEDICAL' class of The KCD:

1. If there are physical symptoms, consult your doctor.
2. If there are NO physical symptoms, consult your doctor.
3. Have a full physical examination and investigations as required.
4. Listen to you body; if you feel something is wrong, you could be right.
5. For existing illnesses, be nice to yourself.
6. Write a 'should' list and work through it as per 'The Mountain Mule.'
7. Create a future that inspires you.
8. Have this positive future subconsciously programmed via NLP, hypnosis, and PS.
9. A mindset of a positive future can be maintained by use of vision boards, mantras, and meditations.
10. Medication use for those where depression has become severe.
11. Ensure excellent nutrition.
12. Consider looking at psychological causes of illness with help of counselor or CBT.

Name the actions you can undertake, that are specific to the class or classes of depression in The KCD that you belong to.
What actions can you take to make this happen?
What is your next step?
What exercise options are available?
What actions can you take to make this happen?
What is your next step?
Where in your life do you feel that there is love?
Who can you give your gratitude and love to?
What actions can you take to increase love in your life?
Name 5 personal positive attributes.
What is your next step?

B. Non-specific measures

1. Purpose

I believe that all human beings have an individual purpose in life. This may be from discovering a new antibiotic to being a mother. It is not the perceived size of the purpose that matters, but the passion and happiness it brings to that person. This life intention has you jumping out of bed, excited about the day. In many cases, this project has no logical reason to exist and may feel impossible to achieve. However, it is in the 'doing' that the happiness comes. If each day you take a step further on the road, however small, positive energy will flow though your body. If you continue to wonder what your purpose is, then answer these questions:

What would you do if you had all the money in the world?

What did you consistently want to do as a child?

What activities do you do that you are so absorbed in, that 4 hours feels like 5 minutes?

If you had a magic wand, what would you being doing now?

What were you doing when you were the happiest you have ever been?

Good fortune and happiness often accompanies following 'your purpose.' Do not despair if you feel it is too late or difficult to achieve. To highlight this, I wish to introduce you to a 50 year old lady, who feels that being a doctor was her purpose. Her name is Ruth and it is unlikely that she will ever go to medical school. However, she looked closely at what being a doctor meant to her. It was the helping and the healing of others. So she began working as a volunteer in a hospice once a week. Ruth enjoyed this so much that she did a course in NLP. She has now begun helping many others and feels her passion is being met.

1. Purpose
What is your purpose?
What actions can you take to make this happen?
What is your next step?

2. Exercise and movement

Exercise is incredibly important for both physical and psychological health. It promotes good fluid circulation around the body, aids in metabolism, increases flexibility, allows release of 'feel good' brain chemicals (endorphins), reduces the risk of many diseases including heart attacks and diabetes, and in many cases maintains a happy mood.

Exercise can address six key areas of our physical and mental well-being. These are strength, stamina, speed, stretch, smiles, and socializing.

Exercise and movement is best achieved as a daily activity. It should also be safe and fun. If this is new to you, then start slowly, such as going for a walk and then increasing in small increments. If the exercise activity includes others then it will include social interaction.

2. Exercise and Movement
What exercise options are available?
What actions can you take to make this happen?
What is your next step?

3. Love

Being around people that you love and who love you is vital in overcoming depression. In this society, where people often live miles away from family members, severe loneliness is extremely common. Even if the relationship between family members is poor, spending a small amount of time in their company can be beneficial.

Showing gratitude and love for friends and family members can remind an individual of how much love there really is. There may be all the love required for a person, but if unexpressed, the feeling of love may be elusive. To get the love we require from others, we sometimes have to make the first move. Therefore, expressing your own love and appreciation of close friends and family may be the first step in receiving the love you deserve.

Love of self is also important. People often respond to an individual in the same way they respond to themselves. In other words, if you cannot love yourself why should someone else? Depression often results in a false sense of low self worth. Telling yourself that you are lovable, even if it feels like a lie, is good practice. You may also list all positive aspects about yourself. Discuss with friends or family what they think about you. If they all think you are great and you disagree, the chances are that you are wrong.

3. Love
Where in your life do you feel that there is love?
Who can you give your gratitude and love to?
What actions can you take to increase love in your life?
Name five personal positive attributes.
What is your next step?

4. Personal growth

If we are not growing as human beings, then we are contracting. For learning is an important aspect of good mental health. It does not matter what the growth is, as long as it is happening. This growth can be studying a course in university, watching interesting documentaries, or learning to shoot baskets on a court. Having the social aspect can often help in the fun of an activity, and in reducing any feelings of loneliness.

4. Personal Growth
What personal growth could you do?
What actions can you take to make this happen?
What is your next step?

5. Touch

Touch and intimacy are vital parts of being human. For the skin is an important organ of emotion. It has billions of touch receptors for hot, cold, pressure, and pain. By stimulating these receptors a cascade of 'feel good' hormones is released in the brain.

Hugging loved ones in particular has been shown to release these important hormones in human beings. Increasing touch with a partner may increase self worth and calm both individuals.

Other ways of increasing touch include having a massage, rubbing lotion into your own skin, and stroking yourself. Touching silk petals of plants and stroking animals are also excellent ways of stimulating skin receptors.

5. Touch
With whom can you increase touch, such as hugging?
What actions can you take to increase your stimulation of skin receptors?
What is your next step?

6. Nature

Nature can significantly rejuvenate the human spirit. There is a frenetic energy to city life, where the majority of the Western world lives. This energy, or vibration, affects all of us. Either we block that energy, or absorb it, and become part of it. Either way it is difficult to remain in a relaxed state. This stress can have a serious effect on a person's mood.

The opposite can be said of the countryside and nature. There is a relaxing energy that trees, plants, mountains, and streams give off. Being around this 'vibration' can have a calming and healing affect on a human being.

Some scientists have suggested that by being able to see the horizon, which occurs at the coast or from a mountain, makes humans feel safe. Our primeval brain wishes to know that there are no enemies around.

I recommend taking a trip away from cities at least once a month, and spending time in a garden or park at least once a week. Also important natural factors include: visiting the coast as often as possible; devoting time to being around animals; ensuring your living environment has natural furniture; and having plants and water features around the home.

6. Nature
What parks or natural spaces are near to you?
Where is your nearest coast and countryside?
What actions can you take to make nature part of your life?
What is your next step?

7. Sleep

See 'Sleep' in Chapter 20, 'Guide to helpful processes and therapeutic substances.'

7. Sleep
What is impairing the quality of your sleep?
What actions can you take to help your sleep?
What is your next step?

8. Foods that love us

As discussed earlier in the chapter on nutrition and depression, food can have a significant effect on our moods.

There are foods that create cravings, such as sugary and fatty foods. These often have a negative effect on mood, whereas good natural foods, such as salads, nuts, seeds, and fruits can improve mood.

It is important to eat plenty of fresh fruit and vegetables in order to absorb enough vitamins, minerals, and anti-oxidants to ensure our health. Supplements can also help. I highly recommend reading Patrick Holford's book 'The Optimum Nutrition Bible: The Book You Have to Read if You Care about Your Health.'

8. Foods that love us
What foods are you craving?
How many pieces of fruit and vegetables do you eat a day?
What would be a good diet for you?
What is your next step?

9. Water

Our bodies require water to maintain a good blood pressure, to help in getting rid of toxins, in production of energy, and to help us keep cool. It is vital that enough fluids are consumed a day to allow good kidney function. The darker the urine, the more dehydrated you are likely to be. Many clinicians suggest at least 2 liters of non-alcoholic fluids per day. Eating a large amount of fruits may mean that you can reduce this amount.

9. Water
How much water do you drink per day?
Is your urine usually dark or light?
How can you start drinking enough fluid?
What is your next step?

10. Sunlight

Sunlight is important in maintaining a happy mood. With lack of adequate light a condition known as Seasonal Affective Disorder (SAD) can occur. There is no exact amount of sunlight that is known to treat SAD. In my experience, a good half an hour minimum in the summer and at least an hour to two in the winter months could be extremely beneficial. If unable to do this or if symptoms still occur then 'light boxes' can be used. These can be of varying strengths but in general 10,000 lux output has been shown to be beneficial.

10. Sunlight
Do you get low in the winter months?
How much time do you spend outdoors?
Are your lights bright enough at work and home?
How can you improve your natural light at work and home?
What is your next step?

11. Good breathing pattern

Breathing allows oxygen to enter our bodies and carbon dioxide to leave. If our breathing is chronically too fast, then it can result in loss of 'too much carbon dioxide.' When this happens the body becomes more acidic. This acidity is thought to cause damage to our organs. As well as this, a poor breathing pattern can increase stress levels. Therefore, learning to reduce and to control breathing rate can help depression.

There are many processes that teach slow and conscious breathing, from the Alexander Technique, to many forms of yoga. You can practice slowing your own breathing down by inspiring 3 seconds, holding for 3 seconds and then expiring for 3 seconds. As you breathe in blow your abdomen out.

11. Good breathing pattern
Do you hyperventilate?
Which actions may help to slow your breathing?
What is your next step?

191

12. Gratitude

Having 'an attitude of gratitude' is fundamental for happiness. For when people look at their lives, there is always something positive to focus on. When we focus on the good, however small, our minds become accustomed to it. The more positive our minds become, the better our mood. I suggest writing a gratitude list at least once a day.

12. Gratitude	
What are 5 things or people that you are grateful for?	*1*
	2
	3
	4
	5

13. Fun and laughter

We were not made to be serious all the time. We are here to have fun. Laughter also helps in dispelling a bad mood.

13. Fun and laughter	
What are 5 FUN activities you can do?	*1*
	2
	3
	4
	5
What is your next step in achieving this?	

14. A generous selfless task for another

By doing simple tasks for others, we are also contributing to ourselves. Firstly, by helping others we take our thoughts away from ourselves, and allow a better perspective on 'our troubles.' Secondly, as human beings are sociable creatures, they are rewarded with a positive mood by helping others.

14. A generous selfless task to another		
What are 5 ways that you can help others?	*1*	
	2	
	3	
	4	
	5	
What is your next step in achieving this?		

15. Socializing

'No man is an Island', said John Donne. 'If I am an Island, I am part of an Island chain,' mentioned the fictional character 'Will' in the hilarious Nick Hornby book 'About a Boy.' When we belong to a collection of people, be it family, work, a club, or a town, we know that we are not alone. Therefore, joining community projects, clubs, or joining friends together can have a positive effect on mood.

15. Socializing
What clubs or community projects can you become involved in?
What actions can you take to make this happen?
What is your next step?

16. Simplifying life

Life can be simple, but tends to get complicated. This can lead to confusion, little time for self, and anxiety. The simpler life is, the more time a person has to enjoy it. Ways of simplifying life include:

Getting rid of 'stuff' you own.

Having a tidy organized home and office.

Have all bills taken care of automatically.

Look at streamlining your spending.

Have good financial planning.

Limit people who are a negative influence on you.

Reduce the daily travel as much as possible.

Co-ordinate with others to get tasks done.

16. Simplifying life
What areas in your life need simplifying?
What actions can you take to make this happen?
What is your next step?

C. Consciousness

It is impossible to be depressed if a person is fully present. For when an individual is in this state of 'full consciousness,' thoughts do not intrude in the sensing of the world. What they see, hear, taste, smell and feel is allowed to flow unimpeded by previous opinions, negativity, or anxiety. There is a relaxation and wonderment, as if the mind is sensing their environment for the first time. When we eat, how much do we actually taste the food? When we look around us, how much are we seeing? In many cases, I feel that it is far healthier to see the same environment with 'new' eyes than to look at a new scene with old ones.

In order to gain increasing consciousness, the following techniques may help:

Do one thing at a time.

Do individual actions slowly and precisely.

Ask yourself what your senses are doing, such as "How does my food taste?" or "What do I see in the scene in front of me?"

Concentrate fully on your breathing.

Breathe slower and deeper.

Laugh deeply and without restriction.

Meditate alone or in a group.

Learn yoga.

Run through your senses in your mind. Ask yourself "What do I see, what do I feel, what do I taste, what do I smell, and what do I hear?"

Learning to be fully conscious will allow an individual to feel connected to him or herself. In many cases it can 'ground them' and take their focus away from thoughts and into the body.

The more relaxed the mind becomes, the easier it will be to put the actions of a happy life into fruition.

Consciousness
What actions can you take to help in becoming present?
How can you make this happen?
What is your next step?

D. Creating your future

Your future is not set, though it probably feels that way. It is not uncommon for the human brain to use past experience and a current mindset to foretell a similar future. However, life is unpredictable. So the truth is, nobody knows what the future will bring. This understanding is fundamental in order to create a happy mind. For people's mood is based more on the future that they think they are about to go into, rather than reality.

It is better for your mood to create a future that you want to happen than to allow your predictions to fill you with dread. Neither positive nor negative futures are 'true,' but the more you focus on one thought pattern, the more likely it is to happen. Having created a picture you like, you can then imagine being there. By using all of your senses of vision, hearing, taste, smell, and feelings, it will become more real in your mind.

When you feel enthused and happy with your potential future, you are more likely to put actions in place to make them happen. The following steps are a simple way of creating your future.

Creating your future
What is your predicted future in the next six months?
Very briefly: how does it make you feel? (Give yourself a mark out of 10)

Now stop
If you could have any predicted future in 6 months, what would it be?
How does this new future make you feel? (Give yourself a mark out of 10)
Has your mood changed by focusing on a positive future?
How do you want your life to be in 1 year?
How do you want your life to be in 5 years?

The next step is to create a vision board. This is a collection of pictures that represent your desired future. This can be done using a large sheet of paper, a pair of scissors, magazines and glue. Alternatively you can make a 'virtual vision board' by downloading pictures on the Internet.
Look at your vision board and imagine that you are there now. What do you?
See
Hear
Feel
Taste
Smell

> *The next step in creating your future is to formulate a mantra. This is a statement that defines how you wish to be or feel, and is not necessarily accurate to your past or present state of mind.*
>
> *Examples include: "I am loved, appreciated, happy and successful." "I am rich and happy."*
>
> *What mantra can you create for yourself?*
>
> *It is useful to look at your vision board daily and to repeat your mantra 10 times a day.*

Notes on creating your future:

1. If you find this difficult, then consider what makes you happy.

2. You can also pretend that you are creating a future for somebody else. It may take away some of the anxiety or emotion that doing it for yourself may cause.

3. You can work on creating your future over weeks, months, or years.

4. This vision is not static and can be changed at any time.

5. Make it fun, get other people involved. You can work on each other's futures.

Chapter 22

Your Daily Plan

'10 simple paths to happiness' is designed to make the process of getting over depression simple. Even though this book covers many issues relating to mood and depression, it all comes down to one thing; that is, putting in a few actions today that will improve your mood and lead you to a happier state. You can concentrate on tomorrow, tomorrow.

Following on from the last chapter, 'Putting it into practice,' **your daily plan** can become your guide to creating a healthy and happy lifestyle. All you need to begin this process is 10–20 minutes per day and a piece of paper.

For every day is like a blank piece of paper. On it, you can write or draw anything that you wish. You can create something new and exciting. Yet, what do most people do? They photocopy yesterday's entries on today's piece of paper, even if they hate those contents. Therefore, each sunrise feels the same. It does not have to be like that. If you change just one thing from the past, then the day will be different. After a few weeks, small regular alterations can accrue to make a better life*.

You choose what goes on your plan. You can add:

1. Contents from yesterday's daily plan.

2. New contents.

3. Structures that work for you daily.

4. Reminders of good fortune in your life and an overall aim in life.

Writing down your daily plan will facilitate your mind in creating a positive life. It can remind you to have fun, be grateful, and to help others. Using the blank reverse of the sheet, you can write down whatever is on your mind. I call this side the 'Splurge Sheet.'

Suggestions for creating and using your day sheet:

You may wish to use my example of a day sheet or create your own. You may download a copy of a day sheet from my website, the address of which is at the end of the book.

1. Have many sheets photocopied with your desired structure and keep them easily available.
2. Fill in the structured side the night before** (this will probably take 10 minutes).
3. When you awake,*** scribble down your thoughts on the reverse side – 'Splurge Sheet.'
4. Cross off each part as you complete the task.
5. Create it after glancing at or studying your vision board or yearly plans.
6. Alter the structure of the sheet at various intervals so that it becomes perfect for you.
7. It is yours and no one else's, so do with it as you wish – you may want to destroy it at the end of the day.
8. When filling in the sheet in the evening, put unfinished tasks from today on the top of your list of actions for tomorrow.****

*What would your life look like, if you did 1000 tasks? Well, that is just five tasks a day for about 6 months.

**By filling in the sheet the night before, your suggested actions will be processed by your subconscious, while you sleep. This will make your plan feel more natural for you to put into action.

***Our mind has many thoughts and most of them are better let out than circulating around the brain. One of the best ways of doing this is to write them down in the morning without thinking about them. It may remind you of something you need to do or just clear the mind for the day ahead. This strategy is illustrated excellently in Julia Cameron's book 'The Artist's Way.' She describes this process as her 'daily sheets'; I call this paper the 'Splurge Sheet.'

**** I was told a story about a life coach who wanted to work for a famous businessman who was going through hard times. He meditated on it, and as 'luck' would have it, bumped into the man at a party one evening. He took this as a positive sign and introduced himself. After chatting for a while, he offered his services, but was declined. Undeterred, the life coach then asked if he could give him a piece of advice, and if it was of value the businessman would send him a check for his services. Six months later, the life coach got a letter saying that his advice had made 10 times the amount in the check. The check was for $10,000. The advice was simple: Write down five of the most important tasks for the day. The most important step would be number 1. However, if by the end of the day not all of the tasks had been completed, those remaining should head the list for the next day.

What you can include on your day sheet

Your daily sheet may be as simple as you wish. Even by writing one or two tasks on it, changes in your life will occur. These tasks will belong to one of the four following categories:

A. Specific measures from The KCD.

B. Non-specific practices that create a happy mood.

C. Consciousness.

D. Creating your future.

NAME:	DATE:

WRITE YOUR MANTRA HERE

A. Specific measures from The KCD

The class or classes of the KCD I am overcoming are?
What is my grade of severity today? /10
Do I need to activate an intervention plan YES/ NO
What are today's KCD actions?

B. Non-specific practices that create a happy mood Choose 3 actions for any of the below subjects.

1. Purpose
2. Exercise and movement
3. Love
4. Personal Growth
5. Touch
6. Nature
7. Sleep
8. Foods that love us
9. Water
10. Good breathing pattern
11. Gratitude – what are 3 things I am grateful for?
12. Fun
13. A generous selfless task to another
14. Socializing
15. Simplifying life

C. Consciousness

What 1 action will you do today to increase your consciousness?
Run through your senses in your mind. Ask yourself what do I see, what do I feel, what do I taste, what do I smell and what do I hear?
Ask yourself what your senses are doing, such as 'how does my food taste?'
Do one thing at a time.
Do individual actions slowly and precisely.
Concentrate fully on your breathing.
Breathe slower and deeper.
Laugh deeply and without restriction.
Meditate alone or in a group.
Learn Yoga.

D. Creating your future What 3 actions today will move me forward in creating the future I want?

203

Helena was not a well-organized person, so committing to writing a daily plan was both a challenge and a blessing. She was suffering from 'The Mountain Mule' class of The KCD, and her inability to say 'NO' to people had led to a cluttered and confusing life.

She was initially worried that a daily plan would take up too much of her time. However, she was pleasantly surprised when the whole process took less than 10 minutes, twice a day. Over the coming weeks and months, she noticed that she had more spare time, even though she was accomplishing greater feats in her life.

She used The KCD format for her plans. An example of one of her completed forms is printed below. In the section entitled 'Specific measures from The KCD,' she wrote down her moods, KCD class, and actions. These consisted of psychotherapy, writing 10 'SHOULDs' per day and saying 'NO' to working late.

When she filled in the area of 'Non-specific practices that create a happy mood,' she focused on fitness, fun, and food. She combined her actions to make the most of her time. For instance, one day a week, she would meet her friend Mary at lunchtime to roller blade in the park, and then they would go to a salad bar together.

In the section on 'consciousness' she would try various activities, from staring at the ducks in the park to deep breathing exercises.

Her future goals included: living by the sea with her children, having an equal loving relationship with a new man, and working as an interior designer. Each day took her at least one step forward. One morning her future actions consisted of printing a list of colleges that did interior design courses. The next, she began to apply for jobs by the coast in Brighton. One task was to find her old CV. The next day she read it. The week after, one of her assignments was to rewrite it.

Helena began to create a routine that really worked for her. When she brushed her teeth, she would tell herself five reasons why she was grateful to be alive. Every morning, she would get up, do 20 sit-ups, drink a glass of water, have an apple and her multivitamins, and would take 15 deep breaths. She would spend a few minutes scribbling in her 'Splurge Sheet,' which included writing down her 'SHOULDs.' Feeling clearer, she would turn over the page and re-read the daily plan that she had completed the night before. Then she would awaken the kids.

The next summer, Helena moved to Brighton and enrolled in a college course for interior design.

NAME: *Helena*   **DATE:** *2 3rd March*

— *I am Loveable*

A. Specific measures from the KC D

Stuggle and the shou[ld]

6/10

NO

psychotherapy 5pm, say No to 3 things

write 10 shoulds

B. Non-specific practices that create a happy mood

Choose 3 actions for any of the below subjects.

1. Purpose
2. Exercise and movement - *rollerblade*
3. Love
4. Personal Growth
5. Touch   12. Fun *football*   c   *kids*
6. Nature *feed duck's with kids*
13. A generous selfless task to another
11. Gratitude – what are 3 things I am grateful for?

7. Sleep
8. Foods that love us
9. Water
10. Good breathing pattern
14. Socializing
15. Simplifying life

C. Consciousness

What 1 action will you do today to increase your consciousness?

Run through your senses in your mind. Ask yourself what do I see, what do I feel, what do I taste, what d[o] smell and what do I hear? *Have a laugh with Marge at work*

Ask yourself what your senses are doing, such as "how does my food taste?"
Do one thing at a time. Do individual actions slowly and precisely. Concentrate fully on your breathing.
Breathe slower and deeper. Laugh deeply and without restriction. Meditate alone or in a group. Learn Yog[a]

D. Creating your future

What 3 actions today will move me forward in creating the future I want?

1 *rewrite CV*   *Finish clearing out garage*   *appt with estate agent*

I feel awful this morning so tired and that I will never get anywhere. That is crazy, I have already sorted out my work and I think I will get that new job, but what if I don't get it. No I am going to be positive, I am going to get it. I am going to imagine having that job. But if I get it, will I have time for the children and will I be good enough. Yes I will make sure I give George and Mary all the time they need and I am good enough. I hate the way my mind works sometimes and ......

Today I feel I should
Be better at work
Sort my mum out all the time
Be thinner
Be younger
Have chosen a better husband
Have more friends
Have a boy friend
Have more money
Go to church more
Be a better dancer
I throw these should away
and get on with my day

As you write your day plan, you may wish to fill in your average mood for the day. A copy of this plan is also available for dow from my website.

Day of the Month

Level	1	2	3	4	5	6	7	8	9	10	11	12	13	14	15	16	17	18	19	20	21	22	23	24	25	26	27	28	29
10																													
9																													
8																													
7																													
6																													
5																													
4																													
3																													
2																													
1																													
	1	2	3	4	5	6	7	8	9	10	11	12	13	14	15	16	17	18	19	20	21	22	23	24	25	26	27	28	29

208

Chapter 23
A Final Few Thoughts

By working through depression, not only will its symptoms reduce in severity and longevity, but also the curtains will be opened on a new way of being. There is no failure for being depressed, only a calling to get better. I believe all depressions, however dark they may be, can be overcome. What is important is for the individual to focus their energy in the right direction. For the more specific a person can be with their treatment, the greater its effectiveness. This was the impetus to create The KCD.

With help from others, belief, and day-to-day actions by the sufferer, the balance can shift from sadness to happiness. That tug of war of life can be won. What is more is that new insights and understandings that have occurred in those dark places often lead to a wiser and more compassionate individual.

Sometimes, when a person's lowest ebb is reached and all seems futile, a massive improvement is about to happen. So, if you feel that you are in that place, then hang on in there and allow yourself the help you deserve. Whatever small positive actions you can take now will make a difference.

The skills that you learn to improve your mood, from depression to a happier state, can propel you even further into a life you may never have imagined. So take heart and keep going. In this way, you can open the curtains on a life that you may have forgotten existed.

THE END.

Quoted and Recommended Books and Websites

1. 'Man's Search for Meaning' by Viktor E. Frankl

2. 'Boundaries: When to Say Yes, When to Say No, to Take Control of Your Life' by H. Cloud and J. Townsend

3. 'British National Formulary (BNF) 63' by Joint Formulary Committee

4. 'The Optimum Nutrition Bible: The Book You Have to Read if You Care about Your Health' by Patrick Holford

5. 'The Artist's Way: A Course in Discovering and Recovering Your Creative Self' by Julia Cameron

6. 'The Depression Cure: The Six-Step Programme to Beat Depression Without Drugs' by Dr Steve Ilardi

7. 'The Depression Cure Formula: 7-Steps to Beat Depression Naturally Now – Exclusive Edition (The Depression and Anxiety Self Help Cure)' by Heather Rose

8. 'DSM-IV-TR: Diagnostic and Statistical Manual of Mental Disorders' by The American Psychiatric Association (31 July 1994)

9. 'The Complete Vision Board Kit' by John Assaraf

10. 'Mantras: Words of Power' by Sivananda Radha

11. 'Be Your Own Life Coach: How to Take Control of Your Life and Achieve Your Wildest Dreams' by Fiona Harrold

12. 'The Essentials Of Psycho-Analysis (Vintage Classics) by Sigmund Freud and Anna Freud

13. 'The Undiscovered Self' by Carl Gustav Jung

14. 'Inner Bonding: Becoming a Loving Parent to Your Inner Child' by Margaret Paul

15. 'The Little CBT Workbook' by Michael Sinclair and Belinda Hollingsworth

16. 'Change Your Thinking with CBT: Overcome Stress, Combat Anxiety and Improve Your Life' by Dr. Sarah Edelman

17. 'Get the Life You Want: The Secrets to Quick & Lasting Life Change' by Richard Bandler and Paul McKenna (Foreword by Paul McKenna) (5 Jan. 2009)

18. 'Richard Bandler's Guide to Trance-formation: Make Your Life Great' (Book and DVD) by Paul Richard Bandler (Foreword by Paul McKenna) (7 Jan. 2010)

19. 'Eye Movement Desensitization and Reprocessing: Basic Principles, Protocols, and Procedures' by Francine Shapiro (11 Oct. 2001)

20. 'The Journey' by Brandon Bays (2003)

21. 'Your Inner Awakening: The Work of Byron Katie: Four Questions That Will Transform Your Life' by Byron Katie

22. 'You Can Heal Your Life' by Louise L. Hay (1 July 2004)

23. On Death and Dying (Scribner Classics) by Elisabeth Kubler-Ross (Jul 2, 1997)

24. 'How to be Idle' by Tom Hodgkinson

http://www.moativationalmedicine.com/
[re illness and psychology]

www.helpguide.org/
[re mental illness]

www.drnickkrasner.com
[re PsychologicalSurgery]

www.primal-page.com/beau.htm
[re Primal Therapy]

211

www.health.com/health/article/0,,20411993_1,00.html   [re supplements]

www.thework.com/

www.thejourney.com/

www.ncbi.nlm.nih.gov/pubmedhealth/PMH0002499/ [re light therapy]

www.nhs.uk/pathways/depression/

www.mind.org.uk/help/diagnoses_and_conditions/depression

www.suicidehotlines.com/national.html [USA]

WWW.THEDEPRESSIONDOCTOR.COM

Lightning Source UK Ltd.
Milton Keynes UK
UKOW050117220213

206648UK00001B/8/P